Praise for *Finish Strong*

"There is no more authoritative or informed individual than Barbara Coombs Lee to lead us in the battle for a peaceful and dignified end-of-life journey. She has been at the forefront since she helped draft the nation's first medical-aid-in-dying law in Oregon. She covers all the issues we must address—from opening the conversations with our families to informing doctors about the kind of care we want at the end of our lives. Read Finish Strong and use it as a guide to consider your own final decisions."

—Diane Rehm, former host and executive producer of
The Diane Rehm Show*, and author of *On My Own

"*Finish Strong* is the kind of book that comes along once in a generation, and Barbara Coombs Lee is nothing short of a historic figure. This book is a game-changing, paradigm-shifting work that will define an inflection point in the way our country thinks about and cares for people who are dying.

"All of us either have a serious illness now or will some time in our future. We will all be called upon to serve as caregivers or care providers. This is a book that every one of us must read, and that we'll all refer to repeatedly over the course of our lifetimes."

—David Muller, M.D., Dean for Medical Education, Icahn School of
Medicine at Mount Sinai in New York

"Barbara Coombs Lee's new book *Finish Strong* will help people who want to pass the gift of life back into the hands of their God thankfully and with dignity. It is a blessing."

—Archbishop Emeritus Desmond Tutu

"*Finish Strong* is the clarion call for the end-of-life choice movement just as *Our Bodies, Ourselves* was for the women's movement. Barbara Coombs Lee's book is an important book, full of candid, helpful advice for people navigating the final stage of their lives."

—Jeanne Phillips, "Dear Abby" advice columnist

"Barbara Coombs Lee gives much-needed guidance on how we can keep our priorities straight as illness advances, helping us approach the end of life without inadvertently getting on a conveyor belt of tests, treatments and misery. *Finish*

Strong serves as a 'field manual' for exploration of autonomy and self-determination in healthcare during the closing years of life."
—Gov. Barbara Roberts, Oregon Governor 1991–95 and author of *Death Without Denial, Grief Without Apology*

"This book is a guide for people who want to help their doctors see them as partners. It's for people who want their doctors to talk to them with candor and kindness and tailor medical treatment to whatever is most important to them in the final chapter of their lives."
—Haider Warraich, M.D., author of *Modern Death: How Medicine Changed the End of Life*

"Adults have the right to decide their own course of treatment at the end of life. Barbara Coombs Lee's wise and compassionate book shows how best to do that."
—Betty Rollin, author of *Last Wish* and *First, You Cry*

"Barbara Coombs Lee's accounts of experiencing a good death in *Finish Strong* include the story of my wife, Brittany Maynard. Brittany's determination to have control over her life's end was possible because of Barbara's advocacy for patients' autonomy and her determination to challenge misguided norms.

"As a society, we need to acknowledge that a positive dying experience should not be left to chance. Barbara shows that it is not something to fear, instead, it's something we should revere. Experiencing a good death is merely the conclusion of a good life."
—Dan Diaz, devoted husband of Brittany Maynard, and advocate for end-of-life options

"*Finish Strong* includes beautiful and powerful stories of people facing the end of life in so many different but strong ways."
—Reverend Alexa Fraser, Unitarian Universalist Congregation of Sterling, Virginia

Finish
Strong

Also by Barbara Coombs Lee

Compassion in Dying: Stories of Dignity and Choice

Finish Strong

Putting **Your** Priorities First at Life's End

Barbara Coombs Lee

compassion
& choices

For quantity purchases of *Finish Strong* or questions for the author, please contact FinishStrongInfo@CompassionAndChoices.org.

Notes:
Some of the names in this book have been changed to pseudonyms.
Internet addresses given in this book were accurate at the time of publication.

Published by Compassion & Choices
8156 S. Wadsworth Blvd., #E-162, Littleton, CO 80128

Printed in the United States of America

Library of Congress Control Number: 20189595599

ISBN
PB: 978-1-7327744-0-7
Ebook: 978-1-7327744-1-4
Audiobook: 978-1-9871926-4-3

Edited by Laura E. Kelly
Book design by Jaye Medalia
Cover image by Naza Abbas Photography
Image of crows, p. 39, © David Vandervoort
Author photo © My Bella Images
See "Notes on Sources" and "Acknowledgments" for other credits

To find out more about *Finish Strong* and Barbara Coombs Lee
visit FinishStrongTheBook.com

To find out more about Compassion & Choices visit CompassionAndChoices.org

Contents

Foreword

A movement is afoot in end-of-life medical care, but doctors are not its leaders. In fact, in their more honest moments, doctors admit they have difficulty finding a balance between medical technology on one hand and living and dying well on the other. Even the most alert and well-intentioned among us at times usher our dying patients onto a conveyor belt of demanding, but potentially futile, treatments and procedures. We should be more humble and let an awareness of mortality, and our patients' priorities, guide our actions. We doctors need help, and Barbara Coombs Lee believes only our patients can deliver that help.

This book is a guide for people who want to help their doctors see them as partners. It's for people who want their doctors to talk to them with candor and kindness and tailor medical treatment to whatever is most important to them in the final chapter of their lives. At first, asking doctors to do this may feel like a journey into the wilderness. But this book is the field manual to turn wilderness exploration into a rewarding adventure. When people venture into the territory of empowered participation in their own healthcare, we doctors are happy to respond.

I first learned of Barbara when I was researching my 2017 book *Modern Death: How Medicine Changed the End of Life*. I wanted to learn about how death, dying and the end of life evolved through the lens of history, science and anthropology. As a physician who was still training at the time of writing the book, I had been trained to think a certain way. One of those ways was to believe that allowing patients to request medication to facilitate their own peaceful dying was wrong and that no physician should ever participate in it. Yet, as I researched and read the stories of those terminally ill patients, who were really the drivers of this movement to reform end-of-life care, I recognized the simple fact that for someone who is dying and suffering, who am I as a physician to make their difficult journey harder? If a patient already has a terminal condition that is going to take their life, who was I to prevent them from at least having some autonomy over how they would like to die?

My research showed that Barbara Coombs Lee, president of Compassion & Choices, a national organization empowering consumers to chart their own course at life's end, was in the forefront of this movement for agency and options at the end of life.

At many points in our lives, all of us are told to stay in our lanes. Entertainers should entertain, actors should act and sports stars should play sports. But it is those who do not heed this call, who break the molds and truly change the world. Barbara Coombs Lee was a nurse who never stayed in her lane, and in doing so, she helped change the world for many many people suffering at the end of life.

Finish Strong is the heartfelt account of a former nurse who often found herself across from patients in the throes of death. Barbara's medical experience means that she can take readers back to earliest days of cardiopulmonary resuscitation (CPR) and paint a vivid image of what medical care was like as it underwent a complete and total revolution, at times for the better, at times for the worse.

While many physicians have written such accounts, Barbara's vantage point is very different. Unlike physicians, who often spend just a few minutes with each patient, nurses come in intimate contact with their patients. Nurses are the ones bathing the patients, watching them gag as they take swathes of pills, and cleaning them multiple times a day. While physicians may perform extensive invasive procedures, it is the nurses who are there with patients as they wake up from the anesthesia, as they take their first steps on the road to what can be a long recovery. Often, patients take their last breaths with only the nurses around.

I learned that eventually Barbara left nursing to practice medicine as a physician assistant and came to perform invasive procedures herself, first in a general medical practice and then as a heart specialist. At a large Veterans Administration Hospital she treated patients both in and out of the hospital and performed coronary angiography. While there, she attended law school at night. So, over several decades Barbara took the heart of a nurse, added a knowledge base in medicine, then the analytic skills of a lawyer. She brought all that into decades of successful advocacy to empower patients and improve medical care. Her perspective, therefore, is invaluable.

Finish Strong goes far beyond a medical memoir to lay out a map for those with elderly loved ones or those who themselves might be approaching an age where death is more than just a hypothetical event beyond the horizon. Building on her decades of experience helping patients and their caregivers navigate the labyrinth that illness traps people in, Barbara's team at Compassion & Choices built a toolkit to help find one's way through. Shared throughout the book, it is a toolkit without a hint of paternalism and a whole lot of kindness.

The first time I actually met Barbara was right before I was about to speak at the Hammer Museum in Los Angeles about my views on patient autonomy. I had heard so much about her, but was unprepared for her warmth and charisma. It seemed fitting that a movement championing a very difficult issue, one that is usually demonized by its opponents, would be led by a woman as compassionate as she is.

It is also fitting to point out that research findings confirm that medical aid in dying, with its fundamental premise of personal agency and autonomy, prompts doctors and other healthcare providers to understand fully what patient-centered care really means. It creates an inherently patient-centric landscape.

Studies suggest that in states where assisted dying is authorized, the quality of end-of-life care for all patients improves, even those who never choose this option. This is because the law fosters open conversations about values and priorities between a dying person, their medical team and their families. The movement has taken some of the issues around death, which were only whispered by patients and caregivers, and brought them into the light. The stigma is gone and people are no longer expected to suffer in silence.

This book does more than just put a much-needed spotlight on the journey toward death and dying. It lights a path of how the best end-of-life experience might be achieved. For readers, it will be the difference between night and day.

Haider Warraich, M.D.
September 2018

Preface

This book offers some of the fruits of my labors in medicine and healthcare advocacy. If you count the years I volunteered as a candy striper under the stern tutelage of the nursing nuns at St. Joseph Hospital in Joliet, Illinois, I've worked in healthcare almost fifty-five years. Dozens of clinical settings and assignments, countless patient encounters, years of advocacy in courtrooms and statehouses, decades of observation and experience—those are the seeds of the fruits borne by these pages.

As a young nurse, intensive care and emergency rooms were my specialty. I loved the blend of high technology and bedside care. I came to believe that comforting attentiveness, clean sheets and a backrub contributed as much to the recovery of frightened and frail patients as all the machinery and medicines did. Still, I was comfortable with the darker side of intensive care, too, inserting large-bore needles into fragile veins, passing tubes down noses and throats to suction or feed, sedating bodies that bolted against the ventilator forcing air into their lungs, tying arms and feet to bedframes when delirious or angry patients thrashed and pulled at their lines. These things were routine and I never questioned them.

So, I can pinpoint exactly when the seed of understanding and passion for a "strong finish" began to germinate. It was with one patient, one night in 1972, as I was on duty in the coronary care unit of Group Health Hospital in Seattle.

Ed had end-stage heart failure. His heart was so weak he was unable to live outside the hospital more than a few weeks before he would decompensate, collect fluid in his lungs, and need to return to our unit for stabilization. Over the months I grew close to Ed and his wife, who often stayed and rubbed Ed's feet until he fell asleep at night. By chance, Ed and I had been photographed together for an article in the Group Health Magazine highlighting the new, state-of-the-art CCU. A copy sat on his bedside table.

One night, Ed slept quietly while I sat at the bank of monitors that formed the nurses' station in the center of the unit. I was watching the sleep of the eight patients on the unit and watching their heart rhythms on the monitors. The electrical activity of Ed's heart became increasingly erratic, so I started into his room to adjust the medication dripping into his vein. I expected to be able to correct this without even waking him up.

Suddenly his heartbeat broke down completely and Ed was in a fatal arrhythmia— ventricular fibrillation. Without hesitation, I did what I was trained to do. I grabbed the defibrillation paddles that hung on the wall, lubricated them quickly, pressed them firmly to Ed's chest and pushed the button. They delivered an electric shock that rocked him in the bed, restored the heart to a normal rhythm and woke Ed up with a cry. He was stunned and angry. "Why did you do that, Barbara?" he shouted. "How dare you? Don't you ever do that to me again!"

I felt terrible, as though I had assaulted him and invaded the sanctity of his body. I apologized and cried. He calmed down and forgave me. The next day Ed left our unit, transferred to a part of the hospital where rescue protocols were not the rule.

Ed taught me that heroics and technological interventions at the end of life are not always what a person wants. But this perspective came as something of a jolt. High-technology medicine was just getting going, with seeming miraculous treatments invented every day. Pacemakers were relatively new on the scene and heart transplants were just becoming feasible. Ventricular assistance devices, implanted defibrillators, a host of complicated tools to monitor heart and lung function and hundreds of procedures and pharmaceutical breakthroughs were rapidly coming online.

In the early 1970s, palliative care was unknown and hospice was in its infancy. When a hospital patient died, it was usually after a long period of "code" activity. The curtains were pulled around the bed, family was excluded, and a bevy of doctors, nurses and trainees cut, poked, pounded, shocked, intubated, passed tubes, connected machines and delivered medication every way possible, including through long needles directly into the heart. Sometimes a doctor would even cut open the chest and massage the heart directly. When all this failed to revive the patient, which was almost always, we broke the sad news to the family and reassured them that "we did everything possible" to save their loved one. Those words were considered to be the kindest, most comforting message at a time of heartbreak and loss.

Twenty years later, high hopes that medical technology would always extend life had begun to fade. Awareness had dawned that a long, drawn out "full code" was just brutal torture of a dying body, and it often left the family traumatized. Now full codes were applied more judiciously, and often more abbreviated if the effort failed to produce results within the first few minutes. Our words of comfort when a person died were just as likely to be "he passed very peacefully." A vision of peace at the end of life had become as treasured as technological wizardry.

But it was not until May 20, 1994, that I heard the words of comfort that seemed to usher in an age when people can find solace in knowing a beloved has completed life on their own terms. That was the day after Jacqueline Kennedy Onassis died of non-Hodgkin's lymphoma. Her son, John F. Kennedy, Jr., emerged from her apartment that morning and comforted the crowd that stood grieving on 5th Avenue. He said, "My mother died surrounded by her friends and her family and her books. She did it in her own way and on her own terms. And we all feel lucky for that."

By the time I heard John Jr. utter those words, the seeds for this book had bloomed into a growing advocacy for just that sort of take-charge attitude in life and death. Jacqueline Kennedy Onassis, seeing death approach, had retreated from the revered towers of the New York Hospital and gone home. She had called those she loved to be with her as she passed quietly, privately from this world. She died with the same grace and dignity with which she lived.

As with any movement, people become motivated when awareness of an injustice breaks into consciousness. The awareness comes as a stunning "Aha!" moment, when you notice suffering and inequality, as if for the first time. You feel energized to find something that averts the suffering, and cures the injustice.

I have often felt that perhaps I worked so hard for public policy to empower people in their healthcare and relieve end-of-life suffering as a kind of redemption for the unnecessary suffering I visited on dying people in my ICU days.

Everyone should have the opportunity to die as Jackie Kennedy did. Everyone should receive candid information and medicine's respectful deference to their beliefs and values. This book aims to deliver that opportunity, through an empowered attitude and the sharing of tools for a more productive doctor-patient relationship. I hope its pages help people with every decision they face about tests or treatments as illness advances and death approaches. I hope it helps people be strong in their understanding and resolve as they apply the final touches to their well-lived lives.

This book is not about medical aid in dying (the option for a terminally ill person to take medication and die peacefully in one's sleep). But as the seeds of change and advocacy have grown over the decades, it so happened that only legal authorization of medical aid in dying has served to break through habits and assumptions perpetuating medical overtreatment and overbearance.

Advance directive laws swept the nation in the 1990s but they were completely ineffective in this regard. The medical establishment, from emergency technicians in ambulances to doctors in hospitals, have ignored advance directives with impunity. Healthcare providers all up and down the line have continued to deliver unnecessary, painful and unwanted treatments to people who had expressed a wish to avoid them when death was imminent. If medical aid in dying seems prominent in my narrative, it is only because it has been the most powerful change agent, and a symbol of the agency and autonomy this book aims for.

Finishing strong will be different for different people. Some will examine their options carefully and decide to dedicate their final months to experimental and taxing treatment. Others may decide to spend precious energy focusing on passing life lessons and values on to their heirs. But for those who choose to "Finish Strong," the common thread will be a certain strength in knowing that treatment decisions were well-considered, and they honored the values and beliefs that gave meaning to the life that is ending.

Barbara Coombs Lee
Portland, Oregon
September 2018

1

An Invitation

Though it has been decades, I still think of Otto.
I may think of him when I drive past a hospital, when I'm stripping a bed, when I feel most vulnerable. I think of him at deathbeds and at funerals. He comes to me with the scent of cigarette smoke and the faint beep of electronic equipment. You could say he haunts me.

I met Otto during my time as a nurse. For more than twenty years, before I went to law school and became a public advocate, I worked in every imaginable clinical setting: as a nurse, a nurse practitioner and a physician assistant.

I did public health on the streets of Harlem. I did night shifts in nursing homes. I did a lot of intensive care and coronary care and spent a lot of time in procedure laboratories and emergency rooms. I rode with EMTs and the fire department in Seattle and administered cardiopulmonary resuscitation (CPR) in unexpected places like the bleachers of football stadiums.

I did witness people die.

Most young Americans are not directly exposed to death on a regular basis. I had a vantage point not accessible to most of my peers. I was struck very early by the vast disparity of these deaths. None of them was easy to witness but some were especially unsettling, and Otto's was perhaps the most unsettling of all. In fact, Otto became an archetype for me—an archetype of the kind of death none of us want.

Otto was in his mid-sixties with advanced emphysema. He was

dark-haired and gaunt, with hooded eyes in a sallow and wasted face. His fingers were stained with nicotine and his shoulders were set in a slump. Before getting sick, he'd been a skilled metal worker in upstate New York. Now he was dying in a teaching hospital in Manhattan.

Otto never had visitors. No friends or family seemed to be in the picture. There were no cards on his nightstand, no flowers on the nearby table. He didn't talk on the telephone, read books or listen to the radio. He didn't even watch television. His one activity was pushing his IV pole down the long hall to the solarium, where he would smoke for hours on end. He didn't have much to say to his caregivers either. Occasionally I'd try to engage him, ask him how he was feeling, invite him to open up. He would answer in monosyllables, if he responded at all.

The man was in agony. His anguish was palpable. His trips to the solarium exhausted him. He was prone to prolonged coughing spells and often lay in bed, gasping for air like a landed fish.

His death was imminent and yet he did not acknowledge this in any way. Indeed, he never seemed to move through the famous five stages that Dr. Elisabeth Kübler-Ross identified as essential to the dying process. He did not get angry. He didn't bargain for a reprieve. And he showed no sign of having arrived at an acceptance of his fate.

Otto made no move to put his affairs in order. He refused to speak to a grief counselor or meet with the chaplain. Despite the severity of his symptoms, his debilitation and his shockingly impoverished life, he clung to his existence the way a cat clings to the trunk of a tree. He remained permanently mired in struggle. He struggled especially to breathe, sweating with the effort, until he exhausted himself, and then he died.

As a young nurse, I was baffled by Otto's attitude. I thought: *What is the deal here? What kind of life is this, and why is it so hard for him to let go of it?* I felt deeply saddened whenever I was around him. And I felt helpless as well. He was a patient whose sharpest suffering was not within our power to diminish.

Several years later, in a Seattle coronary care unit, I met another man whose death became iconic for me. His name was Nate. He was about ten years older than Otto and yet somehow, he looked younger. His straight silver hair swept back from his forehead and his warm dark eyes met mine easily. Before his illness, he'd been a history teacher at a local high school, where he'd remained a vital and popular presence long after most of his peers retired.

He was dying of heart disease and his doctor had the grace to let him die without a lot of heroics or paraphernalia. At the time, heart transplants were not yet a viable option, and they still aren't for people his age. Nate's physician, the chief of cardiology service, was in his seventies himself and had a clear-eyed acceptance of the fact that his patient's death was inevitable and imminent. Moreover, he was unafraid to let his own deep connection to human suffering inform his decisions and guide his practice. He needed no persuasion to do the right thing. Although we had easy access to new state-of-the-art technology, he told us to take Nate off all the machines and let his death come peacefully. So, we did. We removed all the wires and tubes, bathed him and told his family that was stationed outside his room that it was time to come in and bid him farewell.

And this they did. One by one, they came in and sat at his bedside and held his hand and had a final, intimate conversation with him. They told him how much they loved him, how very much he meant to them and how they would carry his memory with them the rest of their days. They promised to tell his story to their children and grandchildren. One of his daughters read him several letters from former students, testifying to how deeply he had influenced their lives. He received all these tributes and loving testimonials with closed eyes and a slight smile. What struck me most during these hours was the equanimity and grace radiating from him, emanating from him to the whole room.

His death, when it came, was just as gentle as a leaf falling from a tree.

Once again, I was bewildered by the story playing out before me. I was as bewildered by Nate's serenity as I had been by Otto's intransigence. I thought: *Now here's a man who has everything to live for! A man wildly beloved by so many. He has a rich and fulfilling life—and look how easily he leaves it.*

After Nate died and we were readying his room for the next patient, putting his belongings in a box, I found a poem by Walter Savage Landor in his nightstand drawer. Its title was "Dying Speech of an Old Philosopher." It was only four lines long:

> *I strove with none, for none was worth my strife.*
> *Nature I loved and, next to Nature, Art:*
> *I warmed both hands before the fire of life;*
> *It sinks, and I am ready to depart.*

I remember standing rooted to the spot, holding that piece of paper with both hands and reading those words over and over again.

I warmed both hands before the fire of life. This, *this* was the vital difference between Nate and Otto. And in that moment, I understood that death is not the terror. Death is not the nightmare hovering at the margins of awareness.

The nightmare, the terror, is never having lived.

We know this unconsciously. I believe that as humans, we have a collective source of unconscious wisdom that comes to us in various forms. Sometimes, as in dreams, it speaks to us in images and metaphors. And I believe this is why many people speak of having approximately the same dream, as follows: It's the last week of school and the day of the final exam. We're about to take a test that's of the utmost importance and we have never attended a single class. We haven't read a page of the textbook, we haven't done any of the coursework or taken a single note. We barely know what this class is about. And yet the final test is upon us.

Dream analysts often interpret this dream as being about life unlived and time misspent. They say it's about our failure to show up, to be present and pay attention to our lives. A momentous event, our death, will someday be upon us and we risk being unprepared. We will be unprepared if we don't take our life assignment

4

seriously and experience the joy and psycho-spiritual growth for which we were born. We will cling desperately to a wasted existence if we do not honor the gift of life by learning to put love and gratitude at its center.

Nursing and the Seeds of Advocacy

Practicing as a clinician showed me time and again how life informs death and death informs life. It showed me the vital importance of being conscious of our mortality and the fragile transience of our precious lives. Approaching the end of life confident of having seized every opportunity for love and kindness seemed to be a primary requirement for a "good" death. Girded with the fullness of a life well-lived, people could die unafraid, as Nate did.

But I also came to see that the field of medicine had a role to play in removing death's sting. It would have to alleviate people's fear of suffering during the dying process. It would have to renounce its habit of aggressive and futile interventions that so often add torture to the experience of dying. After twenty-five years in the medical field, I was spurred by the profound injustices dying patients were forced to endure. I wondered how society might make a transition to less fearsome dying and more compassionate living.

Without any idea of how this quest might take shape, I enrolled in night school at Lewis and Clark's Northwestern College of Law and became versed in its theory and practice. In 1989, I gained admission to the Oregon State Bar. In 1991, after several years of traditional health law practice, I joined the staff of the Oregon Senate Healthcare and Bioethics Committee. As it happened, this was the final year that Oregon State Senator Frank L. Roberts introduced one of the first medical aid-in-dying bills in the nation. (The committee did not approve the bill and, tragically, Senator Roberts died of prostate cancer two years later, suffering precisely the kind of slow and agonizing death he had sought to help Oregonians avoid.)

In 1993, when I read in my church bulletin that a group was

forming to draft an aid-in-dying bill to appear on Oregon's general election ballot, I answered the call. I became one of three chief petitioners who filed the Oregon Death with Dignity Act as a citizens' initiative in 1994. I served as a spokesperson for the issue through two statewide campaigns and spent the next 14 years defending the resulting Death with Dignity law from efforts to undo it in every governmental arena—legislative, executive and judicial. Oregon's law gained no security until 2006, when the U.S Supreme Court finally declared that states do have authority to adopt medical aid in dying as part of the legitimate practice of medicine. Opponents had finally run out of political and legal maneuvers to reverse the expressed will of Oregon voters. Now, 20 years later, attacks on end-of-life choices focus mostly on jurisdictions outside Oregon.

There was no defining moment when I decided to make this advocacy the driving force of my life's work. Rather, one legal challenge surfaced and then another. Each attack seemed so misinformed and misguided that walking away was unthinkable.

And then there was the public response when defenders of Oregon's new law prevailed: the outpouring of gratitude and testimony from the terminally ill. Hearing that thousands of these people finally felt peace of mind and a sense of autonomy over their own fate brought me more professional and personal gratification than I could have imagined.

I knew powerful forces would seek to overturn the law and try to impose their own personal and religious beliefs on others. I couldn't just stand by and watch them wrest this hard-won relief away from patients. Moreover, it had become obvious that authorization of medical aid in dying was having a profound and positive impact on medical treatment. At last we were seeing progress in respect for the wishes of dying patients, the treatment of pain and other agonizing symptoms, and the general quality of end-of-life care. These improvements were extending far beyond the small numbers of patients who requested medication to die peacefully in their sleep.

In 2006, after winning at the Oregon ballot twice, losing then winning in the Oregon legislature, battling federal agencies, surviving two attempts in Congress to nullify Oregon's law and winning two separate cases before the U.S. Supreme Court, Oregon's law finally seemed secure. But there remained much work to do and this is still true. Work goes on to make medical aid in dying accessible to those who need it, to make sure its practice follows the spirit and the letter of the law, and to assist those in other states clamoring to follow Oregon's lead.

In 2008, I also served as a senior adviser for the Washington State Death with Dignity ballot initiative, which voters approved by an 18-point margin. Washington became the second state to authorize medical aid in dying, followed by Montana, Vermont, California, Colorado, the District of Columbia, Hawai'i, New Jersey and Maine.

Educating and Consulting in End-of-Life Decisions

From 1996 to 2018, I had the privilege of serving as President and CEO of the national nonprofit organization Compassion & Choices (C&C) and its predecessor organization, Compassion in Dying. In the last two years I transitioned to President and now serve as President Emerita/Senior Adviser. Today Compassion & Choices fills the vital roles of education and advocacy for end-of-life decisions. Its mission is to improve care, expand options and empower everyone to chart their end-of-life journey. We do this through targeted legislation in states across the U.S., with litigation to clarify or change the law, and public education. We promote an attitude of curiosity about medical tests and treatments, encouraging patients to inquire about how treatments may help and how they may hurt as illness advances. We provide information and support to terminally ill clients and their loved ones and finally, we improve care by establishing this basic principle: To be valid, a medical decision must be fully informed and must reflect the values and priorities of the person it most affects—the patient.

Compassion & Choices has been responsible for several

substantial breakthroughs in public policy. Through a carefully selected lawsuit, C&C established the legal principle that under-treated pain at the end of life is a form of elder abuse. We worked to pass laws in California and New York ensuring that patients who inquire about end-of-life options receive comprehensive and accurate information from their doctors. We sponsored the first law making education in pain and palliative care a requirement for medical licensure renewal.

Though my political and legal work has been different from my clinical work in nearly every way, they are similar in that each has involved intimate dialogue with people in the final stages of their lives. So it would seem—although I never set out to do so—that I've made a lifetime study of how Americans die.

And the truth is that dying in America is a terrible mess.

Maria and Her Son's Cautionary Tale

Just as Otto and Nate became archetypes for me during my time as a clinician, representing, respectively, a bad death and a good one, similar archetypes have emerged during my time as a public advocate. As Otto's story haunts me on a personal level, another story haunts me on a societal level. It has become the archetype of medical treatment gone terribly wrong, resulting in a wretched death.

It's the story of Maria, an impressive and worldly figure in her early eighties. Maria was originally from Argentina, where she ran a secondary school. She radiated the competence, common sense and work ethic that were her defining qualities. She was a woman of stature and intelligence, accustomed to taking on responsibility and savoring a sense of accomplishment. She had raised her family in California and her husband of 50 years died there.

After her husband's death, she continued to live independently as long as she could, with the help of her son, Paco, and his wife, who lived close by. But crippling arthritis and congestive heart failure eventually took their toll and at the age of 81, Maria decided to move into a care center. Upon this transition, she signed forms refusing resuscitation efforts and extraordinary life-sustaining measures if she suffered a medical crisis. Indeed, in 2001, she signed a series of four such forms stating her clear wish not to have resuscitation attempted and not to be treated aggressively if a life-threatening event occurred.

At the age of 82, Maria suffered severe stomach pains that brought her to the emergency room. Mentally, she was as sharp as ever. She brought her medical records with her and she made sure the two physicians who saw her in the emergency room had copies. She made sure they had her advance directives as well.

After Maria was treated and admitted to a medical unit, her family went home. That night, while she slept, the quick and painless death she had planned for came to her. Her heart stopped and she very quietly ceased breathing.

If only this were the end of her story.

Within moments, bedlam overtook this peaceful scene as hospital personnel swung into action to wrest the tranquil death from her. Those attending her called a full code. A team rushed in, shocked her heart back into contractions and attached her to a mechanical ventilator. Then they transferred her to the intensive care unit (ICU).

Paco's phone rang at 2:30 a.m. with the news that his mother's condition had deteriorated. He could hardly believe what he found when he arrived at the hospital. His mother, so determined never to be sustained by machines, was bound like an insect in a complex web of machinery. Tubes ran into her mouth, down her throat and into her lungs. Tubes ran up her nostrils and into her bladder and her veins. Soft straps tied her to the bed so she wouldn't pull at the tubes invading nearly every orifice of her body. Her misery was palpable.

So Paco—poor, shocked Paco—began the difficult process of assessing the situation: How did this happen? What was the extent of his mother's trauma? And what would she want now, after her one true wish had been violated?

Against all odds, Maria had survived this ordeal without brain damage and she was able to communicate with her son by way of hand squeezes: one for yes and two for no. Paco's conversation with his mother went something like this:

"Mom, do you know where you are?"

One squeeze.

"Your heart and breathing stopped and they started them up again. Are you okay with that?"

Two squeezes.

"That's what I thought, Mom. I'm so sorry your wishes were disregarded. Now that you're here though, are you willing to try to recover in the ICU?"

Two squeezes.

"Do you understand you're likely to die if they remove these machines?"

One squeeze.

"Do you still want the machines taken away?"

One squeeze.

"Mom are you saying you'd rather pass on than remain on these machines?"

One long, hard squeeze.

Paco emerged from this conversation with unequivocal clarity. He was a devoted son and the idea of his mother's death filled him with grief but he was determined to do her the honor of restoring her agency and respecting her directives. He approached her team of doctors with this clarity and this determination.

But the doctors had their own ideas. They did not consider Maria competent enough to make her own decisions. They dismissed her hand-squeeze communication as unreliable. And because she had a slim chance of surviving—in whatever compromised state—they felt free to disregard her advance directive, which began, "If I am terminally ill . . ." They ignored the document altogether, ignored her clearly expressed wishes and ignored her son.

Over the next ten days, Paco often found Maria semi-conscious, moaning and writhing in her bed. He asked the nurses and doctors: Why can't you keep my mother comfortable? No one on the staff had answers for him. No one wanted to talk about her end-of-life wishes. Nobody suggested that allowing a natural death—not heroics—might be the appropriate course of action here.

Finally, after many days of clear deterioration, Paco was able to persuade the doctors to remove life support. This conversation took place over the phone and Paco asked that the medical staff wait until he arrived. He wanted to be at his mother's bedside when the breathing support came off.

When he arrived in the ICU an hour later, he found his mother alone in her room. The ventilator and all other equipment had already been removed. Paco was shocked to see her gasping for breath. She was dying, in terror and alone.

Multiple catastrophes occurred here: wrongful resuscitation, failure to honor a person's clearly stated wish, dismissal of an advance directive and inadequate palliative or comfort care. All were avoidable. None could be undone.

Paco wanted to prevent this from happening to others and in 2002, he worked with Compassion & Choices to publicize the case and demand accountability. Ultimately, the State Department of Health did issue a citation to the hospital for violating Maria's rights and failing to honor her requests. But Compassion & Choices' lawsuit—for elder abuse and violation of an advance directive—was thrown out of court. In California, once a person dies, their pain and suffering are no longer "actionable," which means their loved ones have no case. In the eyes of the law, Maria's anguish never happened.

Stories like Maria's remain common across the nation. Too many people die in pain. Too many people suffer needlessly. Too many linger in distress: hands tied down, organs attached to tubes and machines as their stated wishes go unheeded. I'm sorry to report that advance directives are often of no help, even when they are readily available. (Learn more about advance directives in Chapter 2: Talking About Death Won't Kill You.)

Our Nation Can Do Better. We Must Do Better.

In one case, an institution *did* do better—a case that for me has attained archetypal status as a wonderful death. This story, however, includes an ironic twist.

Lorraine Bayless was an 87-year-old woman living in a retirement community called Glenwood Gardens in Bakersfield, California. On February 26, 2013, Bayless collapsed in the dining room of her facility. (Later it would be revealed that she'd suffered a stroke so massive that it shut down all brain function immediately.) As Lorraine lay serenely on the floor, someone on the scene called 9-1-1. Over the phone, a Bakersfield fire dispatcher tried frantically to persuade a staff nurse on site to start CPR.

The nurse refused, saying that Glenwood Gardens' policy did not allow employees to perform CPR on residents. The dispatcher became more aggressive, asking the nurse to hand the phone to any passerby. Again, the nurse refused.

For several minutes, the dispatcher badgered, cajoled and pleaded with the nurse to begin CPR herself or give the phone to someone who would. "Is there anybody that's willing to help this lady and not let her die?" she demanded at one point.

"Not at this time," the nurse told her.

Bayless died swiftly and painlessly on the cafeteria floor that afternoon, though that fact was not acknowledged until she arrived at Mercy Southwest Hospital. And when I speak about her publicly, I often say, "We should all be so lucky."

The ironic twist to this story is that our nation's media presented this death as a travesty of our elder care system. The *New York Times* called the 911 transcript "shocking" and reported that the incident "has raised a chorus of outrage on cable television, talk radio and social media, and vigorous, unanimous condemnation of the nurse, as yet unidentified, and the center where she works."

Indeed, the chorus of outrage was deafening. The entire country, it seemed, was abuzz with sanctimony. Young news anchors opined that 85-year-old women could be physically fit and bounce back easily from total collapse of cardiovascular function. Doctors and ethicists weighed in against the Glenwood facility. The national clamor became a story in itself, garnering high-profile headlines of its own.

All this righteous indignation managed to obscure several important points: First, CPR is seldom a success, especially on the elderly. A staggering 85 percent of those who have resuscitation attempts in the hospital do not survive to be discharged. Patients who need assistance with daily living, who have a range of medical problems or a terminal illness, survive resuscitation attempts in the 0 to 2 percent range. The statistics concerning the elderly are especially daunting. Cardiac arrests outside the hospital carry a survival rate of less than 10 percent among patients in their eighties. Moreover, CPR itself poses a litany of terrible risks: broken ribs and/or fractured sternum, punctured lungs or liver, vomit in the lungs, considerable pain and even brain damage.

Furthermore, survivors often experience sharply reduced quality of life. A major stroke or other catastrophe can result in permanent impairment on every level, physical and cognitive. Most elders live in terror of becoming helpless, demented, incontinent and completely dependent on others for the simplest tasks of daily life. Lorraine Bayless was among them and she did manage to avoid her worst nightmare. She lived independently until her dying moment. She never entered the long and torturous decline so many of her peers endure.

To the surprise of countless people who assumed a lawsuit was a foregone conclusion, the family of Lorraine Bayless did not take issue with her swift and natural death. In a statement released to the public in the wake of the media frenzy, they said:

> "It was our beloved mother and grandmother's wish to die naturally and without any kind of life-prolonging intervention. We understand that the 911 tape of this event has caused concern, but our family knows that mom had full knowledge of the limitations of Glenwood Gardens, and is at peace. We also have no desire, nor is it the nature of our family, to seek legal recourse or try to profit from what is a lesson we can all learn from."

What is the lesson these clear-eyed people considered so self-evident? That life ends. It ends for all of us. If we're lucky, we live life to the fullest into a hearty and advanced age—but not forever. And that irreducible truth remains unalterable, no matter how ardently we seek to ignore it or how much technology we deploy against it.

Lorraine Bayless' story reveals the attitudes and expectations we're up against as a nation. Allowing nature to take its course inspires shock and censure, even when the patient is quite elderly and has requested that any witness to their swift death refrain from intervention. If the medical establishment doesn't succeed in running roughshod over our stated wishes, the rest of the nation gets up in arms when a natural and painless death occurs.

"Why Steep Yourself in Death?"

How we die matters. As physician and author Atul Gawande writes in his landmark 2014 book, *Being Mortal*, "Life has meaning because it is a story. And in stories, endings matter." A good death is one that honors the life that's been lived. I see my life's work today as a quest to help make a good death accessible to everyone. And in keeping with our cultural attitudes toward death, this has struck many of my peers as a morbid preoccupation. On countless occasions, well-intentioned people have asked me, "Why would a healthy, vibrant person like you choose to steep yourself in death?"

My reason is simple. I believe death is an essential and ever-present element of our human condition. I believe living and dying don't fall into a clean binary. Some part of ourselves and our experience dies every day while something else is born. I believe that since ultimately, we cannot run from our own death, we must instead work toward it—during the entire course of our lives. Many have observed that those for whom death is imminent often seem further along in their psychological and spiritual growth. From Mitch Albom's famous book *Tuesdays with Morrie* to political columnist Charles Krauthammer's and John McCain's public announcements of their imminent deaths, popular press, stories and commentaries often bring wisdom and grace from the dying. These people have essential messages for the rest of us.

What are the most pressing requests, concerns and desires of the actively dying? How can we best provide authentic comfort and support to loved ones preparing to cross this final threshold? How can we work toward the best possible final phase of our own lives? We can all benefit from grappling with these questions and bearing intimate witness to the answers—not only at the end of our lives but at this very moment.

The terminally ill people with whom I work want very simple things. They want to avoid suffering. They want effective pain management. They want to remain lucid and engaged with life as long as they possibly can. They want assurance that their treatment decisions are well informed and don't subvert their primary values, priorities and the quality of their remaining months or years. They want options that can allow death to come peacefully when it comes.

When I ask myself why these simple requests are so hard to fulfill, I conclude that it's because Americans desperately want to obscure death's inevitability. Political leaders collude with fundamentalist religious voices to enforce an authoritarian dogma in which death is always the enemy, always to be battled, never to be welcomed and certainly never invited.

In antiquity, stoics like philosopher Epicurus asserted that the art of living well and dying well are one. And of course, the spiritual practices of indigenous peoples honored the cycles of birth and life and death. Today though, many religious leaders renounce acceptance of mortality as indicative of a growing "culture of death," as they themselves claim to represent a "culture of life."

Well, the ancients understood that life and death aren't cultural. They are two aspects of nature. There is no "culture of life" versus a "culture of death," locked in a struggle for dominance. Instead, I see a culture of dogma locked in a struggle with a culture of dignity.

It's an age-old controversy: Those living in the culture of dogma find God's guidance and moral authority in a source outside their own individual conscience. They accept rules from this external source and are encouraged to feel guilt and shame if they do not follow those rules.

Those adhering to a culture of dignity find God—or whatever name they call the transcendent and divine—by looking deep within and their individual conscience is their moral compass. They strive toward an authentic wholeness grounded in love and mystery. They feel, not guilty or ashamed, but empty and destitute if they are not allowed to make authentic decisions from a place of their own personal integrity.

Choices Can Ease the Sting of Death

I meet people from all over the nation as they are preparing to die. They have no time to waste on politics or dogma. Each is putting the finishing touches on their life's adventure and immersing themselves in its truths, its loves, its mysteries. Yes, they are grieving the loss of everything they cherish, including their own earthly existence. But over and over we see how coming into the fullness of their personhood as they die—and having choices about how to die—helps remove the sting of death.

Open and honest communication also eases the sting. When people are finally able to have candid conversation about their wishes for the end-of-life experience, they report feeling an overwhelming relief.

Quite often, however, people feel surrounded by loved ones who cannot accept or acknowledge that the end is near.

"Don't talk like that, Mom. You'll outlive us all."

"Doctors don't know everything. Only God knows what's in store. You have to keep the faith. Keep up the good fight."

"My best friend's mother-in-law had the same thing and was told she'd be gone by Christmas, and now it's twenty years later and she's the picture of perfect health."

We've all heard such entreaties. The people who say them mean well. They have kind intentions. But such evasions serve no one, least of all a dying person who is seeking authenticity and true intimacy during the precious time that remains.

This book aims to dispel that kind of denial and societal censorship. It promotes a brave new model of medical decision-making. It supports candor, curiosity and individual agency. It offers alternatives to the conveyor-belt approach of automatic, futile and burdensome overtreatment. It reminds the reader, over and over, that there is always a choice among treatment options. Statements that we "must" perform some surgery or begin some treatment are never true.

Legacy of the Baby Boomers

During my own youth, sex was the impossible topic; the one people were afraid to mention in polite company. Books like *Our Bodies, Ourselves* and *The Joy of Sex* were positively ground-breaking in their provision of straightforward, matter-of-fact information, aimed at demystifying the subject and empowering readers with knowledge, confidence, agency and choice. They were an early legacy and one of the gifts the baby boomer generation will leave to society as we gradually die out.

We boomers were conceived after World War II and raised in the time of hope and prosperity that began in 1946. I was born in 1947. We are a large demographic and an influential one. As baby boomers moved through significant life stages, we changed every one. Dying will be no different.

Boomers defy convention. Our sense of dominion and agency is so strong some call it self-centeredness. War protest. Mind-altering drugs. Life-altering music, from Woodstock to the Beatles. Civil rights struggles. Natural birthing. End of the draft. The women's movement. These factors and more shaped us into a generation of independents, skeptical of government, comfortable with experimentation and highly individualistic.

These are the characteristics shaping our attitudes as we contemplate elderhood, physical decline and death from terminal illness. We are entering the common age of retirement, age 67, in droves. We bring with us the attitudes, values and habits of a lifetime. We are not likely to retreat now from an attitude of informed agency to one of ignorant submission to authority figures and we wish to pass this torch to subsequent generations, who surely deserve to inherit it.

Americans' blind faith in medical authority—the common idea that doctors know best what tests and treatments are best for us— is about to undergo a sea change. The purpose of this book is to help people navigate and implement that change.

Some of you already believe, or intuitively sense, that people should have better choices at the end of life. I believe we're going through a period similar to the consciousness-raising period of the women's movement. It was a time when all of the injustices—all of the violations of human liberty—had been going on for decades. But suddenly, by the thousands, women came to realizations as they never had before: *This actually isn't right. It's not right that I'm being out-earned by a male co-worker who's less skilled than I am. It's not okay that I put up with my boss patting my backside during my workday. It isn't right that in spite of stellar performance reviews, I get passed over for that promotion.* (In my own case, I was working as a physician assistant when I applied for a job with an orthopedist. He actually said to me, "You'd be great for this job, but I want to hire a man.")

Consciousness and Candor

Awareness dawned in women's individual and collective consciousness. So, it is with the end-of-life issues we've all faced. It's in the recognition of injustice in the experiences we have lived through—the bad deaths, the prolonged agonies, the thwarted desires. These things should not have happened. The people who suffered through them should not have had to suffer through them. And we, who sat by the bedside (perhaps feeling trapped and impotent, unable to do anything for our loved ones) shouldn't have had to feel that way either. Or if we did stand with a loved one who made a decision that invited death to come, we shouldn't have had to shroud that in secrecy. We shouldn't have to feel the societal stigma of guilt and shame. That's an injustice too.

To realize that these are injustices is the first step of end-of-life activism. The second step is to resolve to let curiosity and candor guide decision-making. The fact is that direct and simple questions can make all the difference in the quality of the last precious months of one's life: *Doctor, will this treatment cure me? Will it extend my life? Maybe? Well, what's the likelihood that it will, and by how much? What are the drawbacks? Are there other options? Am I dying? How about the quality of my remaining time? How about comfort care?*

Asking questions and insisting on candor from the doctor sounds intimidating to many people. The first time we do it, we may feel weak and uncertain. But as with a muscle, our ability to do this will strengthen with use. The "candor muscle" can help us have an end-of-life experience our loves ones can take comfort in recalling. It will help our families, like Nate's, savor the privilege of our loving, peaceful passage, and spare others, like Maria's, from tormented memories. But we must take an active part in this process rather than expect our doctors, or anyone else, to initiate it. Throughout this book I offer ideas and scripts for how you can talk to your doctors.

Lest I be misunderstood here, let me state for the record that I know doctors are well-intentioned. I believe that almost always, they're driven by beneficence. By beneficence, I mean the desire to do good for other people and to provide their patients with the best care possible. The problem is that beneficence can morph into paternalism when the professionals delivering care believe they are the only ones in a position to judge what's best for their patients. And when this attitude is institutionalized and there really are no choices besides the ones deemed best by institutional authorities, this paternalism becomes something like oppression.

And finally, when the government gets involved and uses its police power to forbid choices not deemed acceptable by medical institutions, then, to my way of thinking, this systemic oppression becomes dictatorial. As the renowned constitutional scholar Ronald Dworkin has written, "To make someone die in a way others approve, but he believes a horrifying contradiction of his life, is a devastating, odious form of tyranny."

I invite you to join me in resisting this tyranny. May we all come prepared to the ultimate and vital journey. Let us strive to find our way forward with courage, clarity and conviction. Let's clear a path, light the way and enable anyone who so wishes, to finish strong.

What Is "Medical Aid in Dying"?

Medical aid in dying allows terminally ill adults to request and receive a prescription for medication, which they may choose to take, to die peacefully in their sleep. To qualify, they must have a prognosis of six months or less to live, be mentally capable and be able to take the medication themselves, if and when they decide to.

Ten U.S. jurisdictions currently authorize medical aid in dying: California, Colorado, Montana, Oregon, Vermont, Washington state, Hawai'i, Washington, D.C, New Jersey and Maine. The legislation is called by various titles in different jurisdictions: Death with Dignity (Oregon, Montana, Washington, D.C., Maine); the End-of-Life Option(s) (California and Colorado); Patient Choice and Control at End of Life (Vermont); Our Care, Our Choice (Hawai'i), Medical Aid in Dying for the Terminally Ill Act (New Jersey). Proposed laws in other states incorporate the terms "aid in dying" or "medical aid in dying" into the law's title.

Whatever the term, the hallmark of these laws is respect for the agency of the dying person. Through multiple well-tested safeguards, these laws assure that the autonomy and decision-making authority for choosing medical aid in dying rest only with the dying person.

2

Talking About Death Won't Kill You (But It Could Improve Your Life)

Do not go gentle into that good night;
Old age should burn and rave at close of day.
Rage, rage against the dying of the light.

These words from Dylan Thomas' 1951 poem come up often when people talk of life's ending. When I hear them, I can't help but picture an ICU doctor muttering them while performing a tracheotomy or delivering cardiopulmonary resuscitation. If some physicians had their way, no one would go gently, and we would all rave and burn—rage and rage—against the natural end of every earthly life.

I consider it an advance that many patients today are inclined to reject this persistent model of futility and abuse. When asked, most people say they *would* prefer to go gently. Both experience and recent studies teach the most essential thing a person can do to achieve a gentle departure is simply and bravely to think and talk about it ahead of time. I would add the second most essential thing is to learn how to impose one's values onto every healthcare decision.

But this is harder than it sounds. Societal norms discourage death talk, and people hold deep prejudices against speaking openly about the end of life. Even those able to accept the idea of death are often more preoccupied with putting their financial affairs in order and making arrangements for their remains. People rarely consider how to navigate skillfully through the process of decline, and this omission has unfortunate consequences.

This was certainly true for my own parents. When my mother and father were in their late seventies, they began to consider their mortality in practical terms. They visited a lawyer to organize their assets and finances, filled out standard advance directive forms and gave instructions to my sister and me.

But as is true for most people, their most specific instructions were about what to do *after* they died. My mother prepared a list of music she wanted at her memorial. They let us know they wanted cremation rather than burial. If one died first, we were to save the ashes and eventually mix them with those of the other, because they wanted their remains co-mingled for eternity. The instructions ended there, so we were left to figure out what they would most like us to do with the combined ashes.

The time came in 1998 when both had died. Ultimately, my sister and I picked out a beautiful clay urn and brought it with us to Chicago. At the side of the grave of their most beloved grandparents we poured both temporary ash containers into the urn and mixed them together with our bare hands. We set it to rest between the caskets of their ancestors, with the ashes of their last dog, Bella, encircling the urn.

The Problem with Vague Planning

As far as advance planning, my parents said precious little about the actual process of dying. They spoke of their priorities for their last days or months only in the vaguest terms. They were healthy and vibrant and expected to stay that way. My father's doctor told him he might live to 100 and he took that hopeful speculation to heart. My mom was less optimistic about her longevity.

We did understand from general conversation that neither of them wanted to linger in a state of semi-consciousness or profound deterioration. But they never spoke openly about how to avert that possibility. I think they assumed they would go from healthy and capable to dead in short order, with no intermediate steps. The treacherous shoals between good health and the grave were never acknowledged, let alone planned for.

Their advance directives were no help. My sister and I were appointed joint surrogates, but their living will did not elaborate further within the sparse instructions of the standard form. Yes, it was clear my parents did not want life-sustaining treatments. But those forms deal only with situations of terminal illness or permanent unconsciousness and are useless for anything short of that.

Surrogates, I found out, need instruction on what to do when a person is just confused, or delirious, or rapidly deteriorating with little hope of recovery. They need to know where a person weighs in on the ultimate scale balancing the quantity of life against its quality. My parents provided very little in the way of this kind of guidance. So, like most people whose parents are dying, my sister and I struggled with uncertainty and guilt. There was no way to know whether we were conforming precisely to what they would want.

My father died first. At age 82 he suffered a massive heart attack during minor surgery to remove a polyp from his colon. To my everlasting regret, I was the one who had persuaded him to undergo the procedure. He actually told the oncologist, "I'm doing this against my better judgment." But I wanted him to do everything possible to be cancer-free, so he consented in order to please me.

I received the call at work from a doctor I never met, who told me my father had suffered a heart attack during his procedure. I had practiced cardiology as a physician assistant for ten years and I knew that heart attacks came in many varieties. Like any daughter hearing such news, I wanted to believe the doctor meant a minor heart attack. I tried to get more information from this doctor, but all he would tell me was that my father was in the ICU and I should come there as soon as possible.

When I saw my father in the ICU, he was barely afloat in the wake of cardiac catastrophe. This was clearly not the aftermath of a minor heart attack. Obviously, he had suffered a cardiac arrest and had been revived—to an extent. He lay unconscious with tubes, wires and lines crisscrossing his body and burns from defibrillation paddles covering his chest. No preparation or conversation can protect a person from the pain of seeing a loved one in such a dire condition. And if that loved one were healthy and vibrant just a few hours before, there is no way to prepare for the shock. His advance directive did not even enter my thoughts, because I so wanted him to live! I could only sob at his bedside, pleading, "Daddy, Daddy, please don't go."

The next four days were a nightmare of confusion and grief. I left the hospital to tell my mother and bring her to my home, so we could all be together. My sister flew across the country and the next day we all went back to the hospital. The doctors seemed pessimistic and I didn't understand why. They spoke in vague terms about the gravity of his illness but no one told us clearly and explicitly that his chances of survival were almost nil. No one suggested it was time to consult his advance directive. No one told us he was close to death. So, I continued to ask uninformed questions: *Wasn't there a chance he could recover? Wasn't the part of his heart that was injured (the very bottom) less likely to cause death? Shouldn't we wait to see whether this setback could be surmounted?*

On the third day, his kidneys gave out because his heart wasn't able to pump blood through them. So renal doctors joined his team, inserted more tubes and began dialysis. In desperation I persuaded myself this was a good sign. I thought his kidneys would be supported while his heart was healing. After all, why would they start dialysis if it wouldn't do him any good?

In my shock, grief and sense of culpability for his condition, I simply could not accept that my father was dying. My denial, and the doctors' collusion with it, cost him several days of torturous, futile treatment and the cold fate of dying among strangers. In order for an advance directive to work, doctors have to tell families in no uncertain terms that the condition the patient wished to avoid is at hand. They have to say what no family wants to hear: Life is departing from the patient and no treatment will restore it. Words like these are spoken too infrequently.

My father did briefly regain consciousness, during which he ordered us to go home and get some rest. As we prepared to heed his wish, he hurriedly told my sister and me, "Take care of your mother."

No sooner had we arrived home and tossed in a load of laundry than the call came from the renal doctor. My father had died. "We should have been there," was my first agonized thought. I asked whether they'd tried to resuscitate him, and the doctor said no. With this sudden and irreducible dose of reality, I felt a rush of gratitude and blurted, "Thank you for that."

Now that my father was gone, my mother's mental state deteriorated rapidly—or perhaps my father's presence had compensated for her encroaching dementia and we never noticed the severity of her decline until that point. When she got lost walking the dog and took a week's worth of pills in two days, it was time to move her to an assisted living facility.

In 1997, two years after my father's death, she developed signs of colon cancer. We decided it was time to move her to my home for hospice care. One day she passed a lot of blood into the toilet and I expressed alarm, wondering if she needed a blood transfusion. Her slight smile conveyed both amusement and wisdom as she told me, in a moment of perfect lucidity, that if it were her time to die, it would be okay.

"Maybe okay for you, Mom," I said, "but we're not ready for you to go."

The family gathered and visited her regularly at my home during the next three months. Several times my mother reiterated that she felt accepting of death. And yet, when her discomfort spurred an increase in her pain meds, and that increase led to delirium and stupor, it would have been comforting to have, in writing, her clear advance instructions to simply keep her sedated and comfortable until she died.

At least she did not die alone, as my father had. One night, as I sat vigil during a January ice storm that crippled the city of Portland, her breathing became labored. I called out for my sister, who came quickly. Our mother died in our arms.

If I could turn back time, knowing what I know now, I would press my parents to provide specific directions for their care in the case of a catastrophe or serious illness. If we'd had an explicit plan for a sudden crisis like a heart attack or a stroke, I might have adapted to my father's situation more quickly. I might have pressed the doctors for more concrete information and a candid assessment of his prognosis. If I'd talked with my mother about comfort care and how people under sedation often die from pneumonia and dehydration, I might have been more comfortable myself when her own departure unfolded along this course.

Certainly, these experiences inform my own behavior now. At age 71, I've made sure my family understands my views about futile treatments if medical catastrophe has felled me and the chance of recovery is slim.

A True Upside to End-of-Life Discussions

The beneficial impact of end-of-life discussions is well documented. One large and multi-institutional study was published in *The Archives of Internal Medicine*. It evaluated the quality of life of patients with advanced cancer during the final days of their lives. Those who had discussed end-of-life values and preferences with their doctors suffered significantly less during their last week of life. A considerable reduction in ICU admissions and high-tech interventions accounted for this outcome. Moreover, the patients who had talked with their doctors also incurred less expense than those who had no such conversations and died tethered to life-prolonging tubes and machines.

But an additional finding is certain to be a game-changer in end-of-life care. For all the suffering they inflicted and all the cost they incurred, the tubes and machines actually bought *no* life extension at all. Can you imagine the bitterness of being trapped in an ICU, remote from family and friends, suffering and isolated, well beyond the point of meaningful exchanges ... and still living no longer than those who have chosen comfort care, who have been able to remain at home with their loved ones around them?

A second study of 323 cancer patients corroborated these trends. It revealed that the patients who had end-of-life talks were three times less likely to spend their final week in intensive care, four times less likely to be on breathing machines and six times less likely to receive CPR. The corresponding editorial, published in the *Journal of the American Medical Association*, provided this summary:

"End-of-life discussions are associated with less aggressive medical care near death and earlier hospice referrals. Aggressive care is associated with worse patient quality of life and worse bereavement adjustment."

How Doctors Talking with Patients Became a Political Football

Doctors have long been rewarded for doing tests and treatments, but not for talking with patients. Aware of the perverse incentives of such a system, in 2009, Oregon congressman Earl Blumenauer sponsored an amendment to the health care reform bill before the U.S. Congress. The section in question, titled "Advance Care Planning Consultation," simply directed Medicare to compensate doctors for talking with patients about what kind of care they would wish for at the end of life.

Blumenauer was confident his proposal would benefit many of society's most vulnerable citizens. He knew that poor and minority patients were the least likely to have such conversations with their physicians. He noted the irony of Medicare's priorities—its willingness to spend untold millions on aggressive and senseless treatments paired with its reluctance to put a few dollars toward end-of-life discussions in the doctor's office.

Blumenauer's amendment had bipartisan support. Its main co-sponsor was Charles Boustany of Louisiana, a Republican doctor who reportedly told Blumenauer that as a cardiovascular surgeon, he'd had many conversations with patients and their families only after it was too late to prevent non-beneficial treatments. He wished they had taken place when there was time for proper reflection, rather than when surgery was upon them.

The amendment also had the backing of a varied coalition, including Catholic Health Systems, the American Association of Retired Persons (AARP), and the American College of Physicians. Initially, it looked like one of those rare proposals that bridged the usual divide between progressive and conservative, red and blue. It called for nothing more than reimbursing doctors for an important medical dialogue.

As Blumenauer put it, "This is a smart and just thing to do for families going through a tough time. Who wouldn't want to know: Can I stay in my home or will I need to move to a hospital or nursing home at some point? What are different treatment options as my health declines? Will I be in pain and what are the side effects of medication?"

During the extensive "mark-up session" of the health care bill in the House Ways and Means Committee, no opposition emerged to Blumenauer's amendment—not a single critique of its language nor a word spoken against its content.

Then a political personality named Betsy McCaughey emerged on the scene. McCaughey was a former lieutenant governor of New York who'd worked to sabotage the Clinton healthcare reform initiatives in the mid 1990s. In a 2009 radio interview, she spoke blatant untruths about this reimbursement provision in the health care bill. She declared that it "would make mandatory, absolutely require, that every five years people in Medicare have a required counseling session that will tell them how to end their life sooner."

Like a children's game of Telephone, this outright lie got repeated and embellished as it made its way along the right-wing pundit brigade. Soon it had become "Mandatory counseling for all seniors at a minimum of every five years, more often if the senior citizen is sick or in a nursing home," as Rush Limbaugh told his millions of listeners a week later. He went on to add, "We can't have counseling for mothers who are thinking of terminating their pregnancy, but we can go in there and counsel people about to die!"

Conservative commentators warned that Blumenauer's provision cleared a path leading straight to federally-sanctioned euthanasia. They speculated that with its passage, the elderly would soon be put to death by the government. The distortions reached a ludicrous low when then–Vice Presidential candidate Sarah Palin referred on her Facebook page to the "death panels" this bill would create. On August 7, 2009, she posted, "The America I know and love is not one in which my parents or my baby with Down Syndrome will have to stand in front of Obama's 'death panel' so his bureaucrats can decide, based on a subjective judgment of their 'level of productivity in society,' whether they are worthy of health care. Such a system is downright evil."

That did the whole thing in.

Across the country, town hall meetings descended into pandemonium as the proposal was hijacked by the hard right. Blumenauer recalled later that some of these town hall participants even told politicians to "keep government out of their Medicare"— which, he noted, would be difficult to pull off since Medicare is, in its entirety, a program of the federal government.

Jim Dau, a spokesman for the AARP, reported that the organization fielded thousands of phone calls in response to the confusion. There was widespread alarm as people believed the bill would require all Medicare recipients to choose a way to die, even if they were healthy.

Though Dau, Blumenauer and fact-checking websites like PolitiFact.com did their best to dispel these ludicrous untruths, the damage was done. Supporters were forced to concede that battle, hoping that in time we would win the war.

During the next six years, the "death panel" hysteria waned while study after study confirmed the benefits of conversations about end-of-life wishes. In 2014, the Institute of Medicine (IOM) vindicated Blumenauer and all his supporters in a report. "Individuals should have time with their doctors to talk about end-of-life issues, and clinicians should receive the training and financial incentives for such discussions," said David Walker, the former comptroller general of the United States and co-chair of the IOM committee that issued the report. And finally, Medicare announced that starting January 1, 2016, it would indeed pay doctors a fee to talk with their patients about end-of-life care.

It's painful to revisit the setbacks endured on the road to informed end-of-life decisions. I devoutly hope you'll let this eventual victory serve you and your loved ones. Talk with your family and your doctor about "what if" scenarios. Let them know where *you* find the balance between the quantity of life and its quality. Talk about how you personally define "quality." (See a sample letter in the next section.)

One of our medical directors had genuine concerns about serving as her father's health care proxy and how to define his quality of life. When he told her that he would be happy with the quality of his life if he were still able to play video games, she felt enormously reassured to have a clear guideline. We offer more conversation starters below.

Starting a Conversation with Your Doctor

Conversations about the end-of-life were not part of standard medical care in my parents' day. If either of them ever talked with their doctors about their wishes for treatment toward the end of life, they never mentioned it to me. It's most likely my father did not, given his goal of living to 100.

I suspect my mother never talked with her doctor about specific wishes either. It was a rare piece of luck that her doctor's medical attitude was more holistic than procedure-driven. When, at age 85, my mother's symptoms and blood tests indicated bowel cancer with metastases to the liver, her doctor made a hospice referral without ever suggesting chemotherapy or surgery.

While I wish upon every reader similar good luck in the final phase of life, I would implore you not to rely on it. Begin this all-important conversation with your own physician soon. Keep in mind, though, that your doctor will probably wait for *you* to broach the subject.

Talking About Your Priorities Early and Often

It is never too early to discuss values and priorities related to advanced illness and the end of life. This is true even for people who have no illness at all. The earlier your loved ones and your doctor hear what is important to you, and the more they hear you repeat it, the more they will be inclined to support you in your decisions and carry them out if you can no longer speak for yourself.

• Make a clear statement about the balance between the quality of life and the absolute quantity of life. This will be a touchstone for every decision about tests or treatments.

• Ground your quality/quantity balance and your priorities in your religious and/or spiritual beliefs. How are they consistent with the beliefs and practices that have given your life meaning? Clarifying this gives your ideas weight and authenticity.

• Create a document, audio recording or video to communicate your philosophy and serve as evidence that your ideas are firm and long-standing. This documentation will make everyone more comfortable if you decide to forego a treatment or stop one that is sustaining your life, like kidney dialysis. (See the "Creating a Video Supplement to Your Advance Directive" box at the end of Chapter 8.)

• Advance directives cover only very specific circumstances, permanent unconsciousness or terminal illness, and very specific life-sustaining treatments like ventilators and feeding tubes. Your healthcare proxy will benefit greatly from more information than an advance directive.

• For the possibility that you decide to cease burdensome treatments, or if you decide to stop eating and drinking, state in your supplementary documents that you would be willing to undergo a psychological examination. Having a mental health professional validate you are making a rational decision will be a great comfort to your doctor and your family. Be sure the therapist is not making a moral judgment but evaluating decision-making ability, because that is the crucial question.

• Give a copy of these documents or recording to several people whom you love and trust, and who are likely to be present if a medical catastrophe occurs.

Maybe you're wondering how to approach the topic without seeming morbid. If you're unsure how to begin this conversation, here are several openers you might consider:

> "I just read about a study that found all that high technology at the end of life doesn't work and just causes suffering. Are you aware that I wouldn't want that?"

> "A friend of mine recently had a terrible death, hooked up to tubes and machines. I think I'd just want to be home with my family. What do you think about a decision like that?"

> "I love so much about my life—being active, spending quality time with my family. If none of that were possible anymore, I'd like to go out peacefully, without a lot of heroics. Does that fit with your medical ethics?"

If you're uncomfortable broaching the topic in person with your doctor, you might want to test the waters with a letter. As a template, you are welcome to use the following "Letter to My Doctor." You may alter it as you wish or leave it as is, to be mailed or hand-delivered to your doctor at your next appointment. (Please note that this letter—created in Oregon—refers to medical aid in dying as an authorized option; if your state does not yet allow for this, you'll want to cut the two paragraphs that invoke it, shown in brackets.)

> Dear Dr. _____,

> It is important to me to stay as healthy and active as possible over the course of my life and to receive excellent and compassionate medical care.

> At the end of life, my personal values and beliefs lead me to want treatment to alleviate suffering and, most important, to ensure that if death becomes inevitable and imminent, it is peaceful for me and my family.

> If there are measures available that may extend my

life, I would like to know the chance and duration of success, and their impact on the quality of my life. If I choose to decline those measures, I ask for your continued support.

If my medical condition becomes incurable and death the only predictable outcome, I would prefer not to suffer, but rather to die in a humane and dignified manner. I would like your reassurance that:

If I am able to speak for myself, my wishes will be honored. If not, the requests from my health care representative and advance directives will be honored.

You will make a referral to hospice as soon as I am eligible should I, or my health care representative, request it.

You will honor my wishes about artificial nutrition and hydration at the onset of permanent unconsciousness or advanced dementia.

You will support me with all options for a gentle death if I become terminally ill.

[As you know, by law Oregonians may ask their physicians for aid in dying, and physicians may provide life-ending medication for mentally competent, terminally ill patients to self-administer at a time of their choosing, without fear of government interference or prosecution.

I don't know if I would ever ingest such medication, but it would give me peace of mind and comfort to have that option. I would like your assurance that you would be able to provide a prescription for aid in dying in the appropriate situation. I am not requesting that you do anything unethical while I am in your care, but I hope for your reassurance that you would eventually support my personal beliefs and end-of-life choices as listed above.]

I hope you will accept this statement as a fully considered decision and an expression of my deeply held views. If you feel you would not be able to honor my requests, please let me know now, while I am able to make choices about my care based on that knowledge.

Signed,

———————————————

This letter and other sample communications can be found at CompassionAndChoices.org/endoflifeplanning.

Finding a True Partner in Your Doctor

Whatever method you choose, your foray into this conversation will be revelatory. If your physician's response reveals that he or she is seriously out of sync with your values and beliefs, this is your cue to find another whom you feel you can trust to honor your wishes. The end of life is no time to find out your core beliefs and those of your doctor are incompatible.

If you do find yourself in search of a new doctor, know that certain distinguishing characteristics are non-negotiable if you are to have a true partnership. The first and perhaps most essential of these qualities is **humanity**. Your physician should be committed to treating you, the person, and not simply your disease.

Don't deal with doctors who take a conveyor belt approach to medicine, prescribing the same protocol to every patient. Don't waste valuable time and energy with blanket assumptions and tunnel-vision. Find someone willing to partner with you in planning your treatment—someone ultimately willing to defer to your priorities and preferences.

Early in my training at New York Hospital, I had the good fortune to witness the genius and humanity of Dr. Fred Plum, a giant in the history of neurological diagnosis and medical teaching. What made him great was his extraordinary skill in tethering his clinical brilliance to the service of humanity. Seeing his interaction with patients remains my most vivid lesson in how kindness

Finding a "Partner Doctor"

Below are some questions you can use to determine if your physician has the humanity, deference and candor to be a good partner to you as you manage a serious or advancing illness.

Does your doctor have **humanity**?

- How do you factor in my priorities, values and goals before recommending a treatment? Do you find a patient's priorities sometimes change over time?

- When would you recommend an invasive procedure or a treatment with difficult side effects? At what point would you not recommend these?

- How will you balance my "quality of life" with debilitating side effects from an aggressive regimen?

Does your doctor show **deference**?

- How do you view the doctor-patient relationship? How do decisions get made?

- Have you ever had a disagreement over treatment with your patient? How would that get resolved if we were to disagree over treatment?

- In terms of your approach, would you say you are more directive or consultative?

- Can you give me an example of your decision-making process with patients?

Is your doctor **candid**?

- If you know that further treatment is probably futile, do you tell your patients this? How?

- If it becomes clear my remaining time is short no matter what we do, I'd like to do less instead of more. Is this something you'd be willing to support?

and compassion are expressed, and how they temper the cruelty of clinical reality.

Each week students of all medical sciences, doctors in training and even other faculty members packed the auditorium for Neurology Grand Rounds. To be assured of a seat, you'd have to get there early.

As Rounds began, Dr. Plum would sit at an oak table at the front of the auditorium. A neurology resident doctor would present a case and describe the presenting symptoms, the course of the illness and results of diagnostic tests. Dr. Plum might ask the resident to expand on some part of the description or ask how the patient responded to this or that test. Then he would rise and call the audience's attention to elements of the presenting symptoms that he found most meaningful. Often these included some obscure, esoteric and seemingly minor sign or symptom, like how the patient's handwriting had changed, or a sensation or smell the patient had started to notice. His affect was authoritative, academic and excited as he elaborated on the symptoms and their significance.

Then he would ask that the patient be escorted into the auditorium, and everything in his affect changed. The focus changed from "a case" to "this person." Dr. Plum slowed his rate of speech, greeted the patient warmly and welcomed him by name. In a gentlemanly fashion, he introduced the people assembled to the patient, never the other way around. He thanked the patient for being willing to teach us about his illness.

Then he asked, very gently, for the patient to respond to questions or demonstrate the bodily dysfunction that provided clues to the nature and location of the tumor or other pathology. Sometimes he helped the patient, with physical support or verbal guidance, to display the limb that didn't move, the word that didn't come or the thought that didn't take shape. He was encouraging and appreciative of their effort. Patients were eager to help, apparently grateful to be truly seen and heard and for the opportunity to help humankind by sharing the details of their frailty with doctors who could learn from it.

Dr. Plum would ask if there were questions from the audience and I saw how others sought to imitate his respect and kindness toward the patient. None, however, came across as compassionate and humane as he.

It was during this same period, my early formative years as a nurse, that I came to appreciate that nurses seem to apply the humane traits of healthcare delivery more easily than physicians. I have tried to cultivate certain characteristics of a nurse's head and a nurse's heart ever since. They have been a help to me—and perhaps will be to you, if you or a loved one are facing an incurable illness.

The first trait is a clear-eyed and resolute willingness to bear witness to human suffering. Nurses don't turn away from suffering, whether it comes in exchange for some gain in health or longevity, for redemption, for love or for no purpose at all.

Second is an empathic attitude, a healing presence broad enough to hold joy and sorrow, rapture and grief. Nurses go to, and stay with, those crossing a threshold, like birth, the throes of recovery or crisis and grief. Nurses reveal ways to accept and cope, ways to heal if cure is not possible. This often means affirming what is sacred in any individual life—living well as long as possible, showing love and honoring human individuality and dignity.

And the third trait is an understanding of the power of human connection. Nurses clasp people's hands, rub their backs or simply hold space for their fear and pain. We know compassion has a human face and that resilience deepens when people do not feel alone. It's the nurse who stays and abides with the person's physical, emotional and psycho-spiritual experience . . . often after the throng of attending doctors leaves the room.

While humanity should be a key distinguishing quality of any healthcare provider, another perhaps harder-to-find attribute of a physician partner is **deference**. When I imagine a doctor with an attitude of humility and respect towards his patients, it brings to mind a dear friend and ally of mine who recently shared his own end-of-life journey with his fellow Oregonians. Dr. Peter

Rasmussen practiced oncology for three decades, and his was a practice of true patient-centeredness in which he routinely deferred to the needs and priorities of those in his care. Having treated cancer patients who suffered terribly in their dying in spite of his skilled palliative treatment, he was a steadfast supporter of Oregon's Death with Dignity law. He helped many of his own cancer patients achieve a gentle death, and he became the doctor to whom his colleagues turned when they had a patient who asked about medical aid in dying. He and I joined forces to educate providers about Oregon's new law and often appeared together before medical conferences. In November of 2014—at the tail end of his own bout with brain cancer—he made use of the law himself.

When Oregon's Death with Dignity law first went into effect in November 1997, a few patients left Peter's practice, saying their disagreement with him on this issue was so profound they felt they could no longer remain in his care. I once heard someone ask Peter what his response had been. Had he tried to persuade these patients to stay? Or had he simply let them go?

Peter replied, "Of course I let them go."

The questioner asked him to explain—why had he said "of course"?

Peter seemed surprised the answer wasn't obvious.

"Because patients are in charge of the doctor-patient relationship," he said.

Patients are in charge of the doctor-patient relationship. This should not be a revolutionary idea, but in our current medical culture, it actually is quite radical. Doctors are still considered formidable authority figures and most people still believe on some level that the doctor is the boss. Physicians, for their part, generally do little to dispel this notion. Even when they pay lip service to "patient-centered care," they do not mean patient-*driven* care. Practically speaking, "patient-centered" can still mean doctors and other providers form a circle around the patient, telling him or her what to do. This simply places the patient at the center of a huddle of external authority.

The new paradigm of shared decision-making calls for physicians who are more collaborative than directive, more consultative than authoritative. For several years I've used an image of crow behavior to help visualize the difference. In the first image, the birds in the circle may think they are being "patient-centered," but the one in the center clearly has no authority. The birds forming the circle mean well. They have benevolent intentions toward the poor bird at the center of their attention. The "centered" one stands anxiously on the receiving end of a lot of scrutiny and opinion and it's clear he's not going to have much to contribute to what gets decided.

The second image is a bird in charge. His posture says he is the ultimate decision-maker. He still receives information and opinion. But he holds his own prize— the values, beliefs and priorities that are important to him. He is still respectful and attentive to the expertise and experience of his advisors. But the discussion

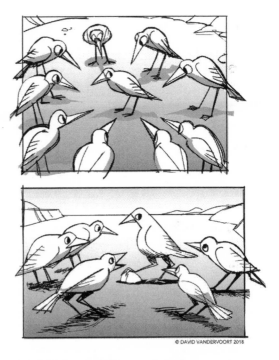

© DAVID VANDERVOORT 2018

is about the fate of the treasure he holds, and he maintains autonomy until the determined course of action meets his approval.

Dr. Rasmussen was ahead of his time. He was wise, and he was right. We are, or should be, in charge of our own health care. Healthcare decisions are about consultation and collaboration, not authority and direction. Find a physician who knows that and forge a relationship in which the trust and dialogue runs both ways. There can be no hope of genuine decision-making and truly informed consent to treatment without that.

Another quality to look for in your partner-doctor is **candor**: The will to level with you about your diagnosis, prognosis and options for care. For many reasons doctors are often reluctant to admit that therapies aimed at curing or slowing progression of a disease have run their course. Understandably, doctors always wish there were more or better treatments to offer, and patients wish this as well. Nevertheless, a time almost always arrives when it is most appropriate to turn to comfort care and efforts to maintain a high quality of life as long as possible. The goal of treatment shifts from "cure" to "care." The dynamic behind reluctance to recognize and accept this shift is complex and deeply embedded in medical education, practice and economics. (We will look at this in more depth in later chapters, particularly Chapter 3: Overtreatment and Diminishing Returns.) Make sure your doctor knows you expect her to level with you if there is little chance that additional treatments will extend life. You might ask about this point-blank: *"If it becomes clear my remaining time is short no matter what we do, I'd like to do less instead of more. Is this something you'd be willing to support?"*

Bottom line: If your doctor does not seem inclined to talk with you from a place of humanity, deference and candor, if he or she prefers "direction" to "collaboration," it may be time to find a more compatible partner.

Discussing Your Wishes with Your Family

As important as it is to speak frankly with your physician, it is equally important to do so with your family. Since there's often little chance the topic will arise naturally, we recommend planning for it. Let your loved ones know you'd like to discuss something important with them. Choose a time and place with care.

At Compassion & Choices, we think Thanksgiving is one ideal time to have a conversation. We like the idea of "talking turkey over turkey." Traditionally Thanksgiving draws several generations of a family to the table. The holiday is relatively relaxed, without the high emotional stakes of Christmas or the New Year.

Nothing more pressing than a hearty dinner and football is on the agenda.

Moreover, the occasion encourages feelings of gratitude. We associate the bounty of the harvest with abundance and well-being. This is a good attitude from which to consider our life story and our deepest desires for the time that remains to us.

Again, if you're at a loss for how to begin, here is one possible opening:

> Mom (or Dad, or Kids), every day I'm so thankful we're all alive and well. And more than anything, I hope we all stay alive and well for a long, long time. But I recently read a book about the importance of talking about the future at a time like this, not despite but because of the fact that everything is good right now.

> The book talked about what most people want toward the end of their lives. Most people want to stay in their homes with as much independence as possible. Most people want friends and family around them and meaningful exchanges with those loved ones. They want to be comfortable, free of pain and aware of their surroundings. But that isn't what most people get, and one reason for this is that they haven't done the groundwork ahead of time. A lot of families begin to consider these questions only in a crisis, which is the worst possible time to make crucial decisions.

> Whatever the future might hold, I want to make sure that your (or my) values and wishes are respected and honored. I want to understand how to protect the rest of our precious time together.

Salespeople are taught to consider common objections to their pitch before coming to the table. We would do well to prepare ourselves for common objections to this conversation before we begin it. The following are the defensive responses you might hear when broaching this emotionally laden topic, as well as some ways to counter them:

"This is a downer. Why think about this depressing stuff?"

RESPONSE: "I love being alive and I admit it's sad to think about life coming to an end. But the knowledge that it will end, as everyone else's will, doesn't depress me. Above all, it makes me appreciate the time I have left and strengthens my resolve to protect its quality at every step."

"I'm perfectly fine and healthy. It isn't yet time to think or talk about death."

RESPONSE: "We plan ahead for every other important event. We don't start planning for retirement the year we stop working. We don't start saving for college when we get our acceptance letter. We recognize these events will be upon us and we begin

Advance Directive Components

An advance directive is a set of documents that "direct" treatment preferences under certain circumstances. Standard advance directives usually include:

- A living will ("what I want")
- Medical durable power of attorney, also called a health care proxy. ("who will speak for me")

Compassion & Choices advises that you consider adding the following documents to your directive to encourage the care you desire:

- **Dementia Provision** (C&C's version) adds language to an advance directive advising physicians and family of your wishes for treatments that could prevent natural death and prolong the period between the onset of advanced dementia and death.

- **Sectarian Healthcare Directive** is an addendum to clarify that your wishes supersede those of any institution's religious policies, and that you wish to be transferred to another facility/sent home if any facility refuses preparing for them decades before. We owe it to ourselves to bring the same forethought to the final phase of life."

"It frightens me to think about dying."

RESPONSE: "I understand that and it's no wonder, given a culture that reinforces mortal fear in every way possible. Today terror and dread dominate conversations about death, even though it's a natural, inevitable and universal part of the circle of life. Even those who rise to overcome fear of dying still must cope with fear of a bad death—one marked by pain, isolation, confusion and suffering. It is this very real, avoidable fear that we can address by planning for a better experience. It eases our fears to know death can be gentle and peaceful for the individual and profoundly meaningful to family and loved ones."

to follow the preferences you've outlined in your advance directive.

• **Hospital Visitation Form** gives unmarried couples hospital visitation authorization.

• **Assisted Living Facility (ALF) Rider** is a contract rider for people who live in assisted-living facilities and would like to stay there until they die. If the facility agrees to include this rider, it will ensure an individual's home is suited to their choices and they will be able to remain in their home to exercise any legal end-of-life option.

• **DNR and POLST**—For individuals in poor health or unlikely to benefit from cardiopulmonary resuscitation efforts, a DNR (Do Not Resuscitate) order and a POLST (Physician Orders for Life-Sustaining Treatment) can give effect to wishes already stated in a directive. That is, they can translate an advance directive (for the future) into a doctor's order (effective in the present) to be followed by emergency medical technicians and other healthcare providers.

Find more information and links to the above documents at CompassionAndChoices.org/endoflifeplanning.

The Role of Advance Directive Forms

Some people might feel tempted to skip the potentially uncomfortable discussions with their family and doctors and just rely on their written advance directive forms to convey their end-of-life care wishes. Those forms cover all the issues, don't they? Hardly. I recommend completing advance directive forms but I do not recommend relying on them alone to avert confusion, settle debates among family members, prevent unnecessary suffering or avoid a prolonged dying process. These forms are just pieces of paper, not truly enforceable as legal documents. They are evidence of your values and your approach to life-sustaining technology when death is imminent. Decisions are made by people, not pieces of paper, and thus the best preparation is people preparation, not paper preparation.

Each state has its own advance directive forms and I recommend using those as a starting place, with addendums to elaborate and clarify as you desire. Those forms will be familiar to healthcare providers in the state, they are free to access and use and usually quite straightforward.

I want to emphasize that it's important that a person's values, priorities and directives be stated consistently to avoid confusion and debate. For that reason, I warn people about one particular advance directive form called "Five Wishes." This form is sold online and advertised as "America's most popular living will," fully valid in 42 states, with more than 30,000,000 copies in circulation.

The "Five Wishes" creators adhere to the philosophical tenet that it is never permissible to intend to end life and thus the form includes an internal inconsistency. It allows a person to decline life-sustaining treatments in certain circumstances, but it also includes an instruction under "What you should keep in mind as my caregiver" that, "I do not want anything done or omitted by my doctors or nurses with the intention of taking my life." This language creates an internal inconsistency in the document and any dissenting physician or family member may claim that to discontinue a machine or treatment that is maintaining life is not allowed, because that action or omission must surely bear the intention of ending life. I recommend crossing out that instruction, initialing and dating the change if you decide to use this particular form.

Finding Your Best Healthcare Proxy

Many families deal with another pitfall, even when candid conversations have taken place. The story of a woman I'll call Greta offers a vivid picture of this potential scenario. Greta came to our attention when her daughter Rae called Compassion & Choices for guidance.

Greta was a retired librarian. Since her husband's death several years earlier, she'd lived alone in the house they had shared for more than four decades. Her two daughters remained within easy visiting distance; Rae was just a few miles away and Leah was about an hour upstate. Their older brother Nathan, however, lived on the opposite coast and saw his mother no more than once a year.

As the town's former librarian, Greta had very close ties in her community. She knew everyone, and everyone knew her. She was a literacy tutor, a pillar of her church and a frequent volunteer at civic events and benefits. Helping others was what kept her going and gave her a daily sense of purpose. She often remarked that the devil would find work for idle hands.

Greta's strong work ethic probably came from growing up on a farm. She was raised with everyday reminders of the cycle of life and death. She was kind and gracious yet unsentimental. She often remarked that when the day came that she could no longer do anything useful, she would know that her time was at hand.

Rae and Leah heard their mother say this often. So, when Greta suffered a massive stroke that left her marginally conscious, they never seriously considered consenting to life-sustaining treatment if there was little hope of their mother regaining mental function. They knew Greta would not want respiratory support, a feeding tube or other forms of artificial sustenance.

Unfortunately, Greta had never thought to formalize her wishes in writing, and her son—the oldest child—was her health-care proxy. Nathan flew into town for the first time in well over a year and would not hear of removing his mother from life support. Though his sisters had spent years faithfully attending to Greta, he now accused them of writing her off and upbraided them for being too quick to "give up on mom."

Some variation of Greta's story occurs often enough to play prominently in the minds of medical providers. Many are acutely aware of what is known as "The Estranged Dissenter," who poses a threat and a risk in decisions about life support. Doctors, nurses and others share a perception that the child least able to let go of a parent on life support is often the one most distant, least involved in that parent's regular life and the one least likely to have been the caregiver. Many presume that guilt over day-to-day absence works as a barrier to accepting imminent death or permanent unconsciousness.

That may be, but as the sibling who was geographically clos-est to my parents, I can say it was shock and grief, not guilt, that made me cling to my father's life support. Without help recognizing how emotions can cloud judgment, a grieving relative can derail a swift and painless death. At their worst, continued denial and unresolved grief can create a drawn-out, ghastly period of artifi-cial maintenance and legal wrangling for months or years.

We can take steps now to avert such a scenario. If you have children with whom you're close both emotionally and geographi-cally and yet your official healthcare proxy is an elder child in a more distant orbit, reassign that crucial role to the child inti-mately aware of your wishes who is willing to honor them. If you're the informal caretaker of an aging parent and you have a distant sibling, explicitly ask to be named the surrogate decision maker. The title of this person varies from state to state. Some call it a "healthcare proxy" and others, an "attorney-in-fact for health-care." But each state has a standard form to appoint this person.

These are available free of charge at the National Hospice and Palliative Care Organization's website at www.caringinfo.org/i4a/pages/index.cfm?pageid=3289.

In Greta's case, resolving this impasse took an intense intervention. Her daughter Rae called a meeting in Greta's home, and together she and her sister Leah confronted their older brother with as much compassion as they could summon. Thinking that guilt played some role in his irrational demands, the sisters strove to assuage his conscience and re-frame the issue for him:

> "Geographic distance might have kept you from visiting as much as you'd have liked, but mom always knew you loved her."

> "Mom told us over and over that she never wanted to be sustained by life support."

> "We know how much you've always cared about doing right by mom. Right now, the way to do right by her is to honor her wishes."

Rae and Leah eventually prevailed. Not everyone is so fortunate. By far the best course of action is to pre-empt such a situation altogether by formally designating a proxy who's promised to protect your priorities, and by making certain every family member who may be involved has heard you talk about your priorities and your desires regarding life-sustaining treatment. This is why we recommend Thanksgiving or some other family gathering for these conversations. This way everyone hears the same thing and if dissent arises, multiple witnesses can reinforce each other. (See also the box "Creating a Video Supplement to Your Advance Directive" on page 166.)

If you do not have a relative or friend willing or able to be your healthcare proxy, you can always try to find an independent professional: a lawyer, especially an elder lawyer, or a geriatric care manager (generally a social worker who specializes in helping seniors manage their care).

It may take some doing to find someone who is willing to take on this job because of uneasiness with the responsibility or even liability concerns. The fee situation would also have to be agreed upon to both parties' satisfaction.

If you were to be incapacitated without having named a surrogate (or proxy), the advance directive statutes in every state except five (Massachusetts, Minnesota, Missouri, Nebraska, and Rhode Island) list individuals, in order, who would have the authority to make decisions. A spouse is the first person designated and the physician is usually last on this list of decision-makers, if there are no close relatives or friends available.

The Limits of an Advance Directive

An advance directive may provide peace of mind by explaining to your doctors and family what healthcare you would prefer to receive if you become incapacitated. But unfortunately, they do little to prevent the kind of futile overtreatment most people wish to avoid. There is increasing understanding that advance directives alone are not enough to ensure that people's end of life goals, priorities and values are honored.

Some of the dismaying reasons why advance directives fall short are outlined below by my colleague and current CEO of Compassion & Choices, Kim Callinan, who wrote a 2016 essay about her grandmother's upsetting death in a hospital.

Reasons advance directives fall short:

• **Limited applicability:** Standard advance directives take effect only when one of two conditions is established: 1) terminal illness and 2) permanent unconsciousness. Confirming that a person is definitely in one of those two categories may take days or weeks, during which time an unwanted hospitalization and much avoidable suffering may have already occurred. The wording of these documents encourages hopeful thinking about forestalling imminent death and restoring absent brain function.

• **Lack of dialogue:** Instructions on a paper are mostly ineffective

Giving Those Around Us the Confidence to Make Hard Decisions

I share these reflections, tips and pitfalls around end-of-life decisions not as someone above the struggle, but as someone who's floundered, made mistakes and suffered in the course of trying to navigate this rocky terrain. I hope by sharing how I fell short of my own ideals in dealing with my parents, you may be spared similar heartache.

Knowing the torture of uncertainty firsthand, I'm committed to

unless the people authorized to give them effect know in advance what the instructions say. The unconscious person and health care proxy often have not discussed the goals, preferences and values outlined in the advance directive. In fact, fewer than three in ten people have actually talked with their loved ones about end-of-life care, according to a survey conducted by the Conversation Project.

• **Lack of relevance:** Since advance directives are, by definition, written in advance—sometimes many years in advance—they often lack relevance to current events and the circumstances in place at the time the documents are needed.

• **Lack of access:** It is all too common that an advance directive along with the DNR order is locked away in a desk or safe when a life-threatening emergency arises, leaving family members and medical providers unsure whether they even exist.

• **Lack of enforcement:** Doctors are not held accountable for following (or not following) advance directives. In fact, most states grant doctors legal protection for either following the instructions in an advance directive or not following them. Until the documents include enforcement mechanisms, physicians have little incentive to follow them. They are more likely to revert to training, to doing everything possible to keep a terminally ill person alive, regardless of whether the treatment only prolongs an agonizing dying process.

preventing it for my own loved ones. Knowing the severe limitations of advance directives, I put my faith in conversations—in having them early and often. My goal is to give those around me the confidence to make hard decisions if they must.

I tell anyone who will listen that if I am unable to respond to them with love and a sound mind, their job is to collaborate with nature to see that my life ends as rapidly as possible. They are not to wait for profound dementia, permanent unconsciousness or terminal illness. An incapacitating stroke, an inability to think and move, delirium, stupor or any serious mental impairment should trigger implementation of my exit strategy.

If seriously compromised mental function is my sorry condition, with slim chance for full recovery, I want everyone to know and agree that I do not want to continue like this. Those in command are to take any opportunity to welcome death's approach. Are there signs of pneumonia or other infection? *Bring it on.* Kidneys underperforming? *Let them falter.* Heart failing or blood pressure falling? *Do nothing.* Not taking in food or water? *So be it.* Any of these circumstances can lead to a gentle, timely death, and my loved ones should treat them as friendly co-conspirators in my demise.

For me, life is thinking and feeling, loving and laughing. It is enjoying nature's beauty and feeling spirit and transcendence around me. If I cannot do these things, and will never do these things, then my life has ended, and the body should follow in short order.

Sometimes my two children, now grown and with families of their own, avert their eyes during these conversations. But my husband and my friends never do. They know what I need most, and they graciously give it to me: the promise to help me finish strong and go gently; the gift of their understanding and loyalty to me, my values and beliefs.

3

Overtreatment and Diminishing Returns

End-of-life care may be the most dramatic example of a phenomenon where, if we actually give people complete information and do what they want, we will spend less money. We would also have a lot less suffering. Indeed, the United States National Academy of Sciences estimated back in 2005 that "between thirty and forty cents of every dollar spent on healthcare is wasted and that amounts to slightly more than a half-trillion dollars a year." It has probably only gotten worse since then.

Our primary concern in this book is not the cost, but rather the enormous and unnecessary harm invasive tests, futile surgeries and toxic medications can cause. Every medical intervention carries a risk of incidental injury and burdensome, sometimes irreversible, side effects. Sometimes those risks are downright catastrophic and can rob us of mental and physical well-being during our final years of life.

Some estimate up to 30 percent of medical treatment is unnecessary, and physicians themselves reported in 2017 that 21 percent of overall care and 25 percent of medical tests are unnecessary. Why has overtreatment become such an expensive and pervasive ill of our system? There are many reasons and I'll list some of them here, with possible strategies for protecting yourself or your loved ones from overtreatment in medical encounters.

Reason #1 for Overtreatment:
Financial Gain

The biggest reason for the tendency to over-treat is our current fee-for-service model of delivering healthcare, in which physicians receive payment, not for curing disease or maintaining health, but for performing tests, procedures and surgeries. Nothing about this traditional payment model rewards good patient outcomes. It simply provides a potent incentive to render a high volume of "services." I don't believe this is a conscious conspiracy or a matter of greed on the part of doctors. I believe it's just the inevitable result of our prevailing medical model, which rewards doing *more* as opposed to doing *better*.

Efforts are underway from policy leaders to move from fee-for-service to values-based payment structures, and these efforts are gradually gaining traction. Health maintenance organizations like Kaiser Permanente have delivered efficient healthcare for decades because their physicians are salaried. The system receives a set payment per enrollee per month instead of payments based on services they deliver. The trend toward paying doctors salaries may be on the rise. Today, highly respected institutions like Cleveland Clinic, Sutter Healthcare, and recently, Geisinger in Pennsylvania, have instituted a system that does not reward doctors financially for "doing more." Nevertheless, we are still a long way from rectifying the perverse incentives of our payment system.

Dr. Leana Wen, a co-author of the 2014 book *When Doctors Don't Listen: How to Avoid Misdiagnoses and Unnecessary Tests*, points out that another regrettable outcome of the fee-for-service system is the natural conflict of interest that arises when doctors receive financial incentives to prioritize one treatment over another.

"When my mother was diagnosed with breast cancer," Dr. Wen writes, "it took her months to find an oncologist she liked. One day, while trying to locate his office number online, she found a listing for him as a highly paid consultant and speaker for a drug—the same chemotherapy drug that he'd put her on. This might have still been the right treatment for her, but it made her wonder and it made her scared. Studies show that as many as 94 percent of doctors report an affiliation with and receive money from drug companies and medical device companies. Though doctors deny these payments influence their decision-making, ample research demonstrates that it does."

Another hard reality of our money-driven system is that care for the elderly suffers from a dearth of options like palliative, hospice and home services, because such offerings don't yield high monetary returns. Preventive measures, or those taken to simply help people have a better quality of life in their elder years, are simply not as profitable as the strenuous interventions that all too often bring misery and suffering.

A final downside of our fee-for-service model is that doctors aren't paid to listen to their patients. Medicare recently approved a modest payment to cover an advance-care planning discussion between patient and doctor, but I doubt the token payment will make much difference. The thorough, in-depth, probing patient interview is largely an experience of the past. Today's appointments tend to be brisk, business-like and bent on efficiency. Several oft-cited studies issued since the 1980s bring the stunning news that American patients usually have between 12 and 18 seconds to tell their doctor what brought them to the appointment before the doctor interrupts them.

Reason #2 for Overtreatment: Doctors' Reluctance to Deliver Bad News

Doctors are as reluctant as the rest of us to face the fact that eventually all lives end. A personal sense of failure and the dread of delivering bad news lead many doctors to keep offering treatments with only the slimmest chance of extending life. All too often these treatments do nothing but compromise the quality of the patient's remaining life (and ironically, can even shorten it through mishap or side effects).

Much has changed in the 50 years since I began my medical

training. Technological testing has largely replaced history-taking and physical examination as the tools of diagnosis. Today, medical education is more likely to focus on teaching listening and communication skills, to make up for the increasing role of technology in patient care. But even when doctors *did* routinely palpate and auscultate, dying patients were the exception. They rarely received the physicians' touch.

During my years as a nurse and then as a physician assistant, I was keenly aware of how rarely death was discussed in a clinical setting. I trained in academic hospitals where teaching rounds took place every morning. An attending doctor led these rounds, and a throng of trainees clustered around the bedside of each patient to ask about symptoms, listen and feel for physical signs of function and dysfunction, generally review the patient's status and formulate a treatment plan.

Each patient, that is, except the ones who were dying. The trainee groups never entered the rooms of such patients and they did not talk about the imminent death. Teaching rounds never included a discussion of end-of-life plans and there was no consideration of these patients' spiritual or emotional needs. It was as though, once a patient was dying, there was nothing worth discovering, evaluating, teaching or discussing. While medical education has improved since I was in school, the reality is that medical professionals still leave medical school largely unprepared to address a patient's final days.

One of the reasons some doctors don't speak candidly about terminal illness is that, despite, or perhaps because of, their frequent proximity to it, they can appear less skillful than non-professionals at dealing with death and moving through grief. Even the field of palliative medicine, which emerged from the arena of hospice and end-of-life care, reinforces our culture's denial of death. Articles and educational forums in palliative care routinely shun words and phrases like "dying," "terminal," or "end of life" in favor of coded ones like "serious disease" and "advanced illness." (See "Chapter 6: Hospice: The Healing Option" for more on palliative care.)

Certainly, doctors need to maintain their professionalism and cannot become overwhelmed by loss and grief. But when doctors become too defended and estranged from their own emotions, their relationships with patients suffer. Dr. Leeat Granek, a critical health psychologist based at Ben-Gurion University in Israel who studies grief and loss, delved into whether oncologists grieve when their patients die. From 2010 to 2011, she conducted a study to determine whether the grief felt by oncologists affected their personal and professional lives. Twenty oncologists of varied age, gender, ethnicity and experience were recruited and interviewed for the study.

Dr. Granek found that "not only do doctors experience grief, but the professional taboo on the emotion also has negative consequences for the doctors themselves, as well as for the quality of care they provide."

Her study revealed that most oncologists suffer from unacknowledged grief, and their sadness is accompanied by feelings of guilt, self-doubt, failure and powerlessness. After a patient's death, oncologists may feel all the symptoms of major depression, such as sadness, emotional withdrawal and a change in mood at home and at work.

Granek's findings also suggest that oncologists feel professional pressure to suppress their grief. This repression and denial can be disastrous for patients since a doctor's bottled-up grief often surfaces as impatience, irritability, exhaustion, inattention and professional cynicism.

Half the study participants admitted their thwarted grief affected the care of subsequent patients. They also reported it spurred them to continue aggressive, fruitless treatments long after palliative care would have been more appropriate, and to distance themselves from patients as death drew near.

Expressed grief is normal and healthy. Danielle Ofri, an associate professor of medicine at New York University School of Medicine and an internist at Bellevue Hospital in New York City, discusses this in her revealing book, *What Doctors Feel: How Emotions Affect the Practice of Medicine*. She explains that both doctors and patients benefit when sadness gets expressed, not suppressed. Suppressed grief threatens mental health and compromises good medical care. It seems clear that doctors' averted grief might play a major role in the irrationally aggressive end-of-life care that is the American standard.

With training and practice, I believe doctors could learn to experience the sadness of a patient's death, acknowledge it, detach it from feelings of guilt or inadequacy, move through it and relate to their patients in a more human and holistic way. A growing number of programs, from those at the University of California in Los Angeles to others at Mount Sinai in New York, are helping doctors do just that.

As I described in Chapter 2, my own father suffered a fatal heart attack at the age of 82. After he died, my sister and I brought my mother to the hospital to see his body before it was taken to the morgue. I have always admired the doctor who came to us in the visitation room, crouched next to my mother's chair, explained what had happened and wept openly.

He didn't know my father well, but he was willing to feel and connect to the universal tragedy of losing one who is most dear. "You are not alone," his tears said to her. "All of us who love deeply must someday bear the pain of loss." An open display of grief and empathy helps us embrace the truth that suffering is the natural response to loss. Such suffering can be one of the most profound experiences in a fully-lived life. This doctor gave my mother a great gift, and even through her encroaching dementia, she never forgot it.

Reason #3 for Overtreatment: Patients' and Families' Expectations

Consumer desires and expectations contribute greatly to doctors' tendency to over-test and over-treat. Often it is the patient's own family members who don't understand or believe that death is imminent—and who are unable to consider any priorities other than delaying death at any cost (in terms of pain and suffering).

I exhibited this desire myself after my father's heart attack. In my shock and fear at seeing him go from healthy to dying in just a few hours, I surely imposed more suffering on him than was necessary. When poor blood flow caused his kidneys to fail, I urged the doctors to begin dialysis. I hoped to buy enough time for his 82-year-old heart to somehow heal. When I am being completely honest, I admit my own remorse factored in the mix as well, since his heart attack happened during a minor surgical procedure I'd persuaded him to undergo.

I know firsthand how hard it is to hear the dire news hidden in a doctor's vague reports and then be the one who authorizes a halt to medical heroics. And I remember how heartbreaking it was to tell my confused and terrified mother that her love of sixty years was gone. In such overwhelming circumstances, people want the comfort of feeling they did everything they could.

Dr. Ken Murray, a retired family practice physician, gained fame in certain circles in 2011 when he published a 2,000-word article titled "How Doctors Die" on Zocalo Public Square, a website affiliated with Arizona State University. In his essay, he pointed out that loved ones often don't understand what it means to ask for "everything." It's all too easy for friends and family to be swept up in the momentum of the crisis and set catastrophe in motion.

"Imagine a scenario," he writes, "in which someone has lost consciousness and been admitted to an emergency room. As is so often the case, no one has made a plan for this situation, and shocked and scared family members find themselves caught up in a maze of choices. They're overwhelmed. When doctors ask if they want 'everything' done, they answer yes. Then the nightmare begins. Sometimes, a family really means, 'do everything,' but often they just mean 'do everything that's reasonable.' The problem is that they may not know what's reasonable—nor, in their confusion and sorrow, will they ask about it or hear what a physician may be telling them. For their part, doctors told to do 'everything' will perform tests, treatments and tortures, whether they are reasonable or not."

The imposition of others' emotional needs upon the dying patient is a very common hazard. Families fear the loss of their loved one and understandably try to avoid the pain of their grief. Sometimes families pressure a patient to accept futile and painful treatments, thinking that's the most loving thing to do. But this is unfair and alienating for the person doing the dying. Patients know best how much suffering they wish to endure and how to make the best of the precious time that's left. Facing death together can bring comfort and courage. Being honest, open and even accepting of an impending death is surely the most difficult thing most people will ever do. But acceptance and support can also be the greatest thing a loving family can give.

Twenty years ago, Dr. David Pisetsky wrote about what he often felt when families asked that he and his team "do everything" to prevent the impending death of their loved one. Fully aware of the futility of medical interventions at such a time, he wrote, "I would like to say, 'Family, only you can do everything. Only you can talk of your love and give kisses before the skin is cold. Only you can talk of the future and of dreams to be fulfilled. Only you can talk of the past when life was resplendent because time seemed infinite.

'Family, only you can oppose the flow of time and enjoy one last day together. Only you can give peace and sustenance for the next journey. Family, only you can do everything. I am only a physician. I can do nothing at all.'"

Reason #4 for Overtreatment: Technology Must Be Utilized

The acquisition of cutting-edge technology in medical settings seems to create an imperative that it be used. Every year the researchers at Dartmouth Atlas Project map the utilization of various technological interventions by geographic location. Cities where ICU beds are bountiful have high per capita rates of ICU admissions. Adding MRI machines increases their per capita use. Supply seems to drive demand, and this is different from every other sector of our economy. Only in healthcare are investments *always* profitable, because merely putting the technology in place will increase demand for it, simply because it's there.

Dr. Daniel Callahan of The Hastings Center, a research institution dedicated to bioethics and the public interest, reports that "new or increased use of medical technology contributes 40 to 50 percent to annual cost increases, and controlling this technology is the most important factor in reducing them." He adds, "An astonishing 40 percent of Americans believe that medical technology can always save their lives; many fewer Europeans share this fantasy. The old joke that Americans believe death is just one more disease to be cured is no longer a joke."

Reason #5 for Overtreatment:
Fear of Lawsuits

According to a national physicians' survey conducted in 2010 by Jackson Healthcare, the nation's third largest healthcare staffing agency, 73 percent of doctors say they order more tests, procedures and treatments than are medically necessary in an effort to prevent lawsuits.

This fear of litigation is vastly exaggerated compared to actual risk. Despite enormous numbers of injuries and fatalities caused by medical error—well over 100,000 per year—patients or their families rarely sue their doctors. Yet doctors feel oppressed by the specter of lawsuits, which can be very stressful and detrimental to a doctor's confidence, if not their career. If a test can rule out the possibility of a problem—no matter how statistically improbable—doctors often decide it's better to be safe than sorry. No one, they rationalize, was ever sued for doing another scan. Many tests are invasive and carry their own risk of complication and injury, but doctors feel safer ordering unnecessary tests than risking accusations of malpractice.

When the most pressing reason for any procedure is protection against a possible lawsuit, the physician is practicing what's known as "defensive medicine." In 2014, Gallup polled healthcare executives on the impact of defensive medicine. The executives' responses revealed that defensive medicine makes up about 26 percent of overall spending on healthcare—about $650 to $850 billion a year. These needless and expensive measures are not, in fact, benign. Every time we consent, we should factor in the risk of harm. How severe are the possible adverse consequences and how likely are they to happen?

Reason #6 for Overtreatment: Comfort Care is Seen as "Giving Up"

Our health care system creates a senseless divide between treatment aimed at curing disease and prolonging life and treatments aimed at providing comfort and improving quality of life. In general, disease-specific treatment and comfort care are offered as an either/or proposition. Patients are told they must relinquish their efforts to survive in order to access the palliative services of hospice. Within this binary system, receiving comfort care has come to mean "giving up."

In August 2010, a study of 151 cancer patients revealed the benefits of doing away with this false dichotomy. Patients with metastatic cancer were randomly assigned to either standard treatment alone, or to early access to palliative care (treatments aimed at providing comfort and improving quality of life), along with standard cancer treatment. Over the course of their advancing illness, the patients with access to palliative care were less likely to choose aggressive treatments like third and fourth line chemotherapy, or be admitted to the ICU—*and yet they lived an average of almost 3 months longer than the standard group.* They also reported better quality of life and experienced less depression.

How to Decide on the Best Medical Plan at End of Life

During the course of every terminal illness, there comes a point of diminishing returns on medical interventions. One treatment may be non-invasive and painless and offer a substantial chance to prolong life. Another may mean an ICU stay, severe discomfort and terrible side effects, while offering little in the way of a longer and better life. The doctors know the difference, and you can know this, too. Only direct questions and answers about the benefits and burdens of each treatment can yield the information patients need to honor their values and make decisions. (For some questions to ask, see the "Having a Say in Your Treatment Plan" box.)

Sometimes the pros and cons of a medical plan, which outlines test recommendations or a specific treatment, can be confusing or unclear. A doctor may list side effects, but it's hard to know whether the list considers your top priorities. For example, maybe blurred vision is a common side effect of a certain medication. This may seem insignificant to the physician, but it will be important to a person for whom reading is their greatest gratification.

Some people simply ask the physician, "What would you do if you were in my place?" Or, "What would you recommend if I were

Having a Say in Your Treatment Plan

Certain illnesses come with certain treatment regimens, but that doesn't mean you have to just accept the standard recommendations. Ask your doctor to specify the risks inherent in any recommended test or treatment and to discuss possible alternatives to it. Carefully consider the downside of any decision. And don't hesitate to ask any of the following questions:

• What's the worst that can happen with this test/treatment? Without it?

• What will happen if we wait? (See Chapter 7: The Secret of Slow Medicine for more on waiting as an option)

• Do we have time to delay this decision?

• Will this test/treatment compromise the quality of the time I have left?

• Is there a comfort care option?

• What course of action would you choose for yourself in my place?

a relative of yours?" If your doctor is among the many who recoil from any hint of a personal exchange, this may lead nowhere useful. But if your question lowers your doctor's defenses and inspires empathy, you may become privy to his or her private assessment of the situation. It is worth asking.

Here are other factors to bear in mind when deciding on medical tests and treatments:

- The phrase "5-year survival rate" means the percentage of patients who are alive five years after receiving the medical test or treatment. What is important is to ask for a comparison of the 5-year survival with and without the recommended test or treatment.

- The phrase *treatment response* (as in "50 percent of patients respond to this treatment") does *not* mean that 50 percent of the people who received this treatment experienced a cure. It means 50 percent of the patients responded to the treatment in some positive way. This could mean 50 percent lived just a few weeks longer than others.

- When a particular treatment extends life in comparison to those who did not receive it, that extension often comes at a cost of pain, debilitation and side effects. Depending on how toxic or invasive the treatment, this cost can be devastating.

- Once a person gets caught up in the momentum of the hospital system, it can be very difficult to avoid an exhaustive and repetitious battery of tests and treatments.

- Comfort care should be an important part of any treatment plan.

- Some treatments for advanced disease are so harsh, they carry a substantial risk of causing death sooner than the disease itself would.

- Pain medications usually affect consciousness and cognitive ability.

- Different diseases cause death in different ways. The only way to learn about symptoms an individual is likely to experience is to ask directly.

Hope is Not a Plan

Our popular culture places a very high premium on hope, but hope can take many forms. Doctors tend to think patients hope for longevity above all else, but a recent poll shows us a different picture.

In 2011, the *National Journal* and the Regence Foundation teamed up to survey Americans about their values and beliefs around end-of-life care. They asked participants to identify the statement that most reflected their beliefs. The overwhelming majority (71 percent) chose, "It is more important to enhance the quality of life for seriously ill patients, even if it means a shorter life." Only 23 percent chose, "It is more important to extend the life of seriously ill patients through every medical intervention possible."

Doctors who believe patients' only desire is to live longer are out of touch with the deeper meaning of hope and healing, which we explore in Chapter 5. Without prompting, doctors rarely ask about the specific hopes of their patients. Nor do they tend to discuss a poor prognosis clearly enough to signal when other hopes should replace the hope for a cure.

Another issue is that often when doctors say a treatment has "a chance of prolonging life," patients will hear that incorrectly, as the possibility of a cure. When the conversation then turns to side effects, such patients may say to themselves, "This treatment may be tough to take. It will make me feel sicker and may cause nausea and fatigue. But as my only hope of a cure, it is worth it." This is why it's often wise for you to repeat back to a doctor what you understand them to have said, in order to avoid any misunderstandings. (For more on this, see "Tips for Combating Overtreatment" box on the next page.)

In a culture that prioritizes "positive thinking" and seeks to keep hope alive at any cost, it might seem cruel to acknowledge, plainly and clearly, that a patient is dying. And yet, to me, it seems far crueler not to do so. No one wants to die prematurely but concentrating on only one kind of hope—the hope for a cure or an extension of life—cheats a dying person out of the chance to make the best decisions and the best use of their valuable time. When doctors reinforce futile hopes at the expense of the truth, they keep dying patients in the dark about their actual prognosis and the scarcity of their remaining time. The danger is that patients nearing the end of life may squander precious days and hours traveling

Tips for Combating Overtreatment

Some tips on how to handle possible reasons you might get put on the "overtreatment conveyor belt."

1. Financial incentives

• Be alert to the varying costs among treatment options.

• Ask if one option would be more or less costly than others.

• Don't be afraid to mention out-of-pocket costs as one factor you would like the doctor to consider.

2. Reluctance to deliver bad news

• Ask outright: "Do you have good news or bad news for me?"

• Acknowledge a doctor's discomfort by saying something like, "It must be hard for you to tell me this."

• Share your preferred communication style with your doctor—candid, gradual or any other—early in the relationship. (Compassion & Choices helps you create your own "Trust Card," designed to help you best connect and communicate with a new specialist, at www.trustcard.org.)

3. My own expectations and my family's

• Don't make decisions quickly, because rapid responses are more likely to arise from emotion than reason.

• Take the time to think about what doctors have shared, talk about it together among family and loved ones and formulate additional questions for clarity, if necessary. Strive for consensus, but know your own values and priorities are most important.

• Keep notes on what you learn about the benefits and burdens of a test or treatment. Refer to these notes before reaching a decision.

to and from a remote cancer center, receiving futile treatments, and feeling too sick to enjoy the love and beauty around them.

Preparing for the Post-Cure Period

Of course, everyone hopes first and foremost to be cured. But when cure is not possible, other priorities rightfully rise in importance—priorities like effective comfort measures, the energy and

4. Available technology

• Ask the crucial questions about *any* test or treatment, whether or not it is offered to you as "the latest thing."

• Ask how long this technology has been available at the facility and about the local experience with it.

• Is there a low-technology means to do the same thing? Why is the new machine or technique better?

5. Defensive medicine

• Ask for specific information about benefits and risks. Ask for more information if it seems incomplete: "Is there anything else I should know before I consent or decline?"

• Ask specifically what will be learned from this test and how that information makes a difference.

• Take responsibility for accepting or declining a test or treatment. "I know there may be a risk in avoiding (or undergoing) this treatment, and I accept that."

6. Negative connotation of "giving up"

• Review your priorities for life's quality and/or duration. Reaffirm what is most important at this time.

• Set goals based on your priorities and promise not to "give up" on your goals. (For example, one goal might be to maintain the strength and energy to visit with loved ones, including grandchildren.)

• Remind yourself what "finishing strong" means to you. Acknowledge the courage and determination you need for this kind of strength.

clarity for meaningful conversations, and the capacity to enjoy what time is left.

Looking ahead to this post-cure period, ask yourself: Do I value extension of life at any cost? Would I forego a slim chance to prolong life for a few months if the treatment made me too sick to enjoy myself? What activities or conditions make life meaningful to me? Is it important to spend the last weeks or months of life at home? Is it a high priority to stay alert for prayer, tender conversations and expressions of love?

Be vigilant about these specific priorities, hopes and wishes that will arise and endure after curative treatments are exhausted. Write them down and share them with your loved ones. Formalize them by simply writing out a document, like a "letter to my loved ones," or make a recording that augments an advance directive. Plan your treatment around protecting these priorities. Make sure your family and your doctors have clarity about what is most important to you.

Above all, it's essential to remember that this is your life, your body and your decision. It's your choice whether and when to halt efforts to prolong life, especially if those efforts come at the expense of your values and priorities. Remember that it is *always* a patient's prerogative to say, "No," to say, "Enough."

In light of all the reasons overtreatment happens—reasons that have nothing to do with our well-being and, in fact, are too often at the expense of it—we must not assume that, "Doctor knows best." We must take care not to comply with a course of action that conflicts with our deepest desires at life's end.

4

Let Me Die Like a Doctor

In the previous chapter, I listed the reasons for modern medical overtreatment in the United States, ending with the recommendation that you question the "doctors know best" adage regarding your own care and personalized medical regimen. When doctors consider undergoing medical treatments themselves, however, it appears they *do* indeed know best. They know how best to die.

A little history here: The modern movement for end-of-life choice traces its roots to a group called The Hemlock Society, which began in California in 1980, moved to Oregon in 1988, and then to Denver in 1995, and changed its name to End-of-Life Choices in 2003. In 2005, End-of-Life Choices merged with Oregon-based Compassion in Dying Federation to form Compassion & Choices (C&C). With a national presence and state-by-state programming and activities, C&C is currently the movement's dominant organization.

In the early days, Hemlock Society members sometimes marched with placards reading *Let Me Die Like A Dog*. The comparison was clear: When a pet is incurably sick and suffering, euthanasia is common and feels like a merciful choice. Yet the comparison was also imperfect and inaccurate. Today's end-of-life choices movement is about individuals making decisions for themselves, after carefully considering various options. It is about autonomy and self-determination, especially in relation to the amount of pain and suffering to be endured. It's not about any other person guessing what a dying person would want and acting based on their own judgment or values, as one would do with a dog or cat. Being entirely patient-driven, medical aid in dying is radically different from euthanasia. Practice standards for medical aid in dying require that the terminally ill individual be mentally competent to make and carry out any request, and that they self-administer the life-ending medication, should they decide to take that final step.

A more accurate slogan for what people are seeking—startling as it might sound—is: *Let Me Die Like A Doctor.*

Die like a doctor? What does that mean? Doctors are not all alike, of course. But doctors tend to plan to die differently than the rest of us. They agree to fewer invasive or aggressive treatments. They choose palliative treatments and suffer less. They don't, themselves, plan to submit to the low-yield and exhaustive gauntlet of tests and interventions they routinely impose on their dying patients.

This revelation took the nation by storm in November 2011 when Dr. Ken Murray, a retired family practice physician, published his article "How Doctors Die," mentioned in the previous chapter. The tagline beneath the article's title read, *It's Not Like the Rest of Us, But It Should Be.*

Dr. Murray wrote of the dramatic disparity that exists between doctors and the general population regarding the last few weeks or months leading up to death. His essay opened with the story of an esteemed colleague and mentor who'd found a lump in his stomach. This orthopedist—called Charlie in the article—consulted a surgeon who found he had pancreatic cancer.

Murray reported that Charlie's surgeon was one of the best in the nation and had developed a surgical technique for pancreatic cancer that could increase a patient's chance of surviving another five years from 5 percent to 15 percent, with some decrease in quality of life. The surgeon could not persuade Charlie to undergo major surgery that carried only a 15 percent chance of helping him. Charlie went home, closed his practice and devoted himself to time with family and to feeling as good as possible. He accepted neither chemotherapy, nor radiation nor surgery. He died at home several months later.

I believe most physicians would call a treatment or surgery with no chance to cure and, at best, a chance to extend the life of only ten people in a hundred "futile." And, if the surgery or treatment itself were risky and painful, with a long recovery time, they would deem it an irrational treatment choice.

But the temptation is so great to offer the dying cutting-edge technology that doctors do not present the treatment to patients as the irrational choice it may be. They present it in such a way that the patient does consent to being cut open, subjected to a long and complicated surgery and assaulted with machines, tubes and drugs for days in an intensive care unit, at enormous financial, emotional and physical cost, for an 85 percent chance of experiencing no benefit.

Murray writes that the only thing such aggressive treatment buys is *misery we would not inflict on a terrorist.* I have witnessed physicians make promises never to inflict futile suffering on each other, should they find themselves in a similar situation as their dying patients. Cease treatment, refrain from resuscitation and treat with opioid analgesics, at home if at all possible.

Murray's article inspired hundreds of comments and swiftly went viral. Several high-profile media venues snapped it up for discussion. London's *Daily Mail* re-printed the article under the provocative headline, *"Why Most Doctors Like Me Would Rather DIE Than Endure the Pain of Treatment We Inflict on Others for Terminal Diseases: Insider Smashes Medicine's Big Taboo."*

But sensationalism aside, there is data to back up Murray's assertion that doctors are likely to resist pointless invasive treatment at the end of life. In 2014, Dr. V.J. Periyakoil, the director of the Stanford Palliative Care Education and Training Program, conducted a study of the attitudes of physicians toward advance directives. A subset of 1,081 doctors completed an advance directive themselves during the course of the survey. Of these respondents, 88.3 percent reported that they would choose a "Do Not

Resuscitate" or "no code" status if they became terminally ill.

Later that year, Dr. Periyakoil unveiled these results at the Annual Scientific Meeting of the American Geriatrics Society. She concluded her presentation with the plaintive questions, "Why do doctors continue to provide high-intensity care for terminally ill patients? Is dying with comfort a best-kept doctors' secret, and why is it that what we provide to patients is different from what we would want for ourselves?"

A second study reflecting this troubling disparity appeared in *The Annals of Internal Medicine* in 2003. In a survey conducted informally at a conference for hospitalists (doctors who work only in hospitals), 98 percent of 250 respondents said that if they had advanced COPD (chronic obstructive pulmonary disease, or emphysema)—which leaves patients in a constant struggle for breath—they would want to be sedated to unconsciousness until they died. Yet, fewer than one percent reported that they had ever offered this option to their COPD patients.

An Ironic Twist

In 2016, researchers at the University of Colorado looking at treatment patterns in 200,000 Medicare beneficiaries found that, in spite of what doctors *say* they would choose at life's end, many actually underwent at least one type of aggressive treatment as often as did people who were not doctors. They found the majority of both groups were hospitalized at least once in the last six months of life, and about the same percentage had a stay in the ICU: 34.6 percent for doctors versus 34.4 percent for non-doctors.

The researchers were surprised at the findings, as they had expected the opposite. They understood their findings as emphasizing just how powerful and persistent is the futile impulse to try and rescue oneself from imminent death. It showed yet again how hard it may be to stop the moving train of technological treatment, even for doctors. On the other hand, the study did show that doctors were more likely to be enrolled in hospice and likely to spend more time in hospice than people who were not doctors.

My own empiric evidence confirms that there is truth to the suspicion that in order to navigate our health system successfully, without ending up in the cycle of overtreatment, it helps to be either a doctor or nurse, be lucky enough to have married one or to have a healthcare proxy who is one.

While we might not all be fortunate enough to be a relative of a doctor or nurse when facing our mortality, I think we can all learn from the actions and pragmatic outlook of healthcare providers in end-of-life situations. These are people who seemed to know the right questions to ask and how to advocate for themselves. They've learned through repeated experience about the limitations of aggressive treatments and modern medicine, and their training and knowledge enable them to perceive when the time has finally come to shift away from hope for long life and toward hope for graceful death.

This book hopes to give you some of those same insights these healthcare providers possess when facing *their* end of life. To inspire you further, I'd like to share a few of their stories.

Forward Looking and Unflinching

Dr. Paul Kalanithi was an extraordinary person by any standard. Paul was 36 when his stage IV lung cancer became apparent. Emerging at the completion of his neurosurgical residency at Stanford, his cancer arrived just as he approached the full bloom of family life and professional accomplishment. No man ever had more to live for.

In the midst of the uncertainty of cancer treatment, Kalanithi and his wife decided to bear a child. For Paul and his wife, Lucy, having a baby was a commitment to live fully and love deeply, precisely *because* he probably would not survive.

In his posthumous 2016 memoir *When Breath Becomes Air*, Paul recounts a decision-making process in which both he and Lucy thought of each other's welfare first. Lucy thought that Paul's choice to spend his precious time as a father should be his. Paul couldn't bear to picture Lucy both husbandless and childless after he died. But, appreciating the enormous caregiving burden for Lucy, he insisted the decision was ultimately hers to make. He recounts,

> "Will having a newborn distract from the time we have together?" she asked. "Don't you think saying goodbye to your child will make your death *more* painful?"

> "Wouldn't it be great if it did?" I said. Lucy and I both felt that life wasn't about avoiding suffering.

> . . . We talked it over. Our families gave their blessing. We decided to have a child. We would carry on living, instead of dying.

Paul died in 2015, and his book publisher asked Lucy Kalanithi to add an epilogue to Paul's memoir. In it she offers this description of the scene at his deathbed,

> He looked at me, his dark eyes alert above the nose bridge of the BiPAP mask, and said clearly, his voice soft but unwavering, 'I'm ready.'" Ready, he meant, to remove the breathing support, to start morphine, to die.

When Breath Becomes Air shot to the top of *The New York Times* bestseller list immediately upon publication in 2016, where it remained for many weeks. Paul Kalanithi's story captivated the nation, not just the tragedy of his untimely death, but the almost impossible generosity with which he accepted it. On her book tour, his wife Lucy sat down with Katie Couric to discuss just how he managed this.

Lucy told Couric, "He'd [long] been interested in this question of how to make a meaningful life and how to face mortality, or to find meaning despite the fact that we're all mortal. Then when he himself was diagnosed with a terminal illness, he did feel ready to face it."

Couric cited the deathbed passage quoted above, in which Paul told his loved ones he was ready to die. Then she asked Lucy whether she herself felt ready in that moment. With emotion, Lucy said that she had been ready as well, and offered this explanation, "He was very ill and for him the most important thing was to be lucid and have mental clarity, so both of us kind of knew that that time was up."

When asked how they could face death so unflinchingly, Lucy cited their medical backgrounds as the source of their brave determination to avoid illusions. Paul and Lucy traveled their paths very much as a team. Whatever they faced, they faced it together. As physicians, Paul and Lucy were able to talk "about what was really happening."

Perhaps no passage of Paul's memoir captures the gratitude and mindfulness of his life and the grace of his exit better than the following paragraph, meant as a message to the daughter he was leaving.

> There is perhaps only one thing to say to this infant, who is all future, overlapping briefly with me, whose life, barring the improbable, is all but past. That message is simple: when you come to one of the many moments in life when you must give an account of yourself, provide a ledger of what you have been, and done, and meant to the world, do not, I pray, discount that you filled a dying man's days with a sated joy, a joy unknown to me in all my prior years, a joy that does not hunger for more and more, but rests, satisfied. In this time, right now, that is an enormous thing.

Paul's lesson to others is to face forthrightly the cards life has dealt you while maintaining an attitude of gratitude and mindfulness for a meaningful ending.

Dying the Way He Lived

This vignette is about maintaining grace in the face of the inevitable. It features my friend from Oregon, Dr. Peter Rasmussen, whom I discussed in Chapter 2 as a model partner-doctor, given his deference to patient-directed care in his oncology practice.

Stricken with glioblastoma in 2014, Peter underwent radiation, chemotherapy and multiple surgeries to stave off the brain tumor's advance. Eventually, when the returns in longevity were outweighed by the price in suffering and inconvenience, he brought those treatments to an end. Peter devoted precious energy during his last year of life to the gracious sharing of his story. He welcomed a journalist from the *Statesman Journal*, the major newspaper published in his town in Oregon, into his home and into his thoughts. He allowed a photographer to capture intimate images of his illness and care. He spoke on camera about the most private aspects of his journey with cancer. Always dedicated to education, he was a teacher to the end.

For eleven months, Peter was a walking testimony to my conviction that a well-lived life provides the best balm for death's sting. When people asked him what he planned to do during what might well be his last six months of life, he told them he didn't believe in

5 Things Doctors Know About End of Life

1. Death is inevitable. Something will be the cause of death for every one of us.

2. We can and should expend great effort to remain healthy, but we should also put some effort into preparing to die well.

3. Medicine has never made a person immortal. All treatment plans will eventually "fail."

4. Keeping these truths in mind is the key to exercising discernment in one of life's most important decisions—when to turn away from futile therapies and focus completely on love, beauty, faith— the things of greatest importance at the close of life.

5. Only the person dying can exercise this discernment, for it arises from their unique experience and life story. Thus, we should respect and honor whatever individuals choose for themselves.

bucket lists. He'd lived his life just as he wanted, in the way that was most meaningful to him.

Although Peter hoped palliative and hospice care would enable him to die naturally, he was comforted knowing he had another option—one which he had fought for on behalf of his own patients years before. In November of 2014, as seizures worsened, and his dying verged on agonal, he made use of medical aid in dying for himself.

After witnessing his last year, I'd say that perhaps Peter's advice to readers looking for a good ending would be to follow his example—simply to press on, with the same values and in the same good life for as long as possible.

Staying Present for Events in Our Lives

I end this chapter by circling back to Dr. Ken Murray and one of his loved ones. Murray concluded his provocative "How Doctors Die" essay with the story of his older cousin Torch, whose lung cancer had spread to his brain. Torch was told that with an aggressive course of treatment—involving three to five chemotherapy sessions a week—he might live four more months. He opted to do none of that. Instead he chose to move in with Murray and enjoy his remaining time—which proved to be twice as long as predicted.

Torch and Murray took a trip to Disneyland, cooked wonderful meals and had a fine time watching sports. Torch was in high spirits during this period. He had no serious pain and eventually he departed from this world quietly, in his sleep. Torch's end-of-life scenario was the one most of us want: at home, mindful, lucid, gentle and steeped in love and appreciation.

Torch didn't want to die, but he knew from his pragmatic, medically-trained cousin that it was even more important not to die badly. He saw the brief amount of time he had left not just as a tragedy but also as an opportunity, and he insisted on making full use of it. In so doing, he illustrated a truth: We can't control the cards we're dealt, but we can decide how to play them.

Precious conversations with loved ones and scenes of reconciliation and joy are only possible when we are conscious, lucid and able to be present for the events happening around us. There are parting gifts we can give and receive from our loved ones during the final phase of our lives, but only if we've made a point of creating and protecting a space where exchanges of this nature can happen.

May we enhance and make the most of our days on earth by being mindful of the fact that they will eventually end. And may we enhance and make the most of our endings by keeping them true to the values of our lives. Or, to put it another way:

May we live fully and well.

And may we die as doctors would choose to die.

5

Hope and Heroism

In America we portray illness, and especially cancer, as an enemy to be conquered. The dominant narrative is one of "fighting" a force that has invaded our bodies, "beating" the occupier and "winning" the battle. A countervailing narrative of graceful surrender to the certainty of death simply does not exist in the prevailing story of aging and illness. Thus, we describe those who die as "losing the battle" with cancer, and always with the silent question of what it would have taken to "win."

A few stories illustrate how this battle metaphor plays out in the U.S., in the media and in real life.

Mixed Messages About a Hero's Good Farewell

Americans always knew Senator John McCain as a war hero. Mere weeks before he died at his Arizona ranch in August 2018, media reports continued to use warrior language to describe his experience with terminal illness. Typical stories included statements like, "As he battles brain cancer and the debilitating side effects of his aggressive treatment . . ." and, "Mr. McCain, 81, is still in the fight, struggling with the grim diagnosis."

Yet the reality was that months before his death, McCain had willingly left behind aggressive surgeries and the ICU so that he could receive a stream of friends at his home, who shared memories with him and his wife. During this time, he enjoyed the beauty of nature around him and carefully chose the speakers for his funeral.

I applaud the less pugilistic media reports about the senator's end-of-life plans. But I had to shake my head when I read a comment in the press from Bob Dole, now 94, who said he planned to tell McCain in an upcoming phone call, "You're a tough guy and you can overcome this." In the conversation I imagined occurring between the two of them, McCain (who had been quoted saying that he now planned "to celebrate with gratitude a life well-lived") gently but firmly set his old friend straight.

Perhaps one of the wisest of McCain's visitors was Senator Joe Biden, who, three years before visiting his dying friend, had very publicly mourned the death of his son, Beau, who died from the same aggressive brain cancer as McCain. Only those two friends would know everything they spoke of during Biden's visit, but Biden leaves no doubt that love and respect—not fighting words—were the main message he wanted to impart.

"I wanted to let him know how much I love him and how much he matters to me and how much I admire his integrity and his courage," Biden told *The New York Times*. Those are the sweet and wise sentiments of one bidding a hero farewell.

A separate *New York Times* article, a tribute column by Timothy Egan written four months before McCain died, also struck a more realistic tone in describing McCain's peaceful and purposeful last days. "McCain is not just plotting the details of his own funeral but living it," wrote Egan in "As He Lay Dying." "He's lucky. Most of us don't get the chance to tell friends and family members how much we love them, to put things in order—and in return, to hear from those people about what a difference a life made to them." Egan also mentioned how McCain's end days reminded him of his mother's, "After we realized that further chemotherapy would just be cosmetic, and add pain to her final days, she chose the McCain route—reflection, planning, settling of personal accounts."

It seems fitting that something termed "the McCain route," the end-of-life story of a Vietnam veteran and long-serving U.S. Senator, is such a positive representation of the sort of heroic, valiant farewell that I describe throughout this chapter.

The Trouble with Medicine's Metaphors

Not long ago, *The Atlantic* published an article titled "The Trouble with Medicine's Metaphors" by Dr. Dhruv Khullar of Massachusetts General Hospital. It discussed the negative effects of militaristic language on the emotional well-being of patients, as demonstrated in multiple studies. Dr. Khullar cites another physician, Zbigniew Lipowski, who studied how patients characterize their illnesses. At the time of diagnosis, patients may view their illness as a challenge, a value, an enemy, a loss or as something else. Follow-up studies indicate those who view their disease as an enemy tend to have higher levels of depression and anxiety, and report a lower quality of life than those who attach a neutral or more positive descriptor to their illness.

Cancer survivor Heather Lagemann says, "While I understand why people use these terms, and I have even spoken them myself, these 'battle' terms make me uncomfortable ... While I was in the midst of cancer treatment—and stripped down to my rawest state, physically and emotionally—people would often tell me to 'keep fighting' or that I would 'beat this.' I was a 'warrior' ... What they didn't seem to understand was that, by saying those things, they were insinuating that the outcome was up to me. That if I 'have what it takes' (whatever that is), I could 'win.' It seemed to be my personal responsibility to cure my own cancer. I was either going to be a winner or a loser."

According to the "battle" narrative, we need two things in order to be victorious in our "fight" against disease or illness. First, we need courage and the will to wage war and persist through multiple battles. In order to prevail against cancer in particular, we need to muster a single-minded focus, a mighty endurance and a high tolerance for suffering. These are to be our primary weapons during painful, debilitating treatments that may go on for years.

Second, we need hope—hope that medical treatment will achieve a total cure and postpone death indefinitely. Irrespective of evidence to the contrary, every impulse is to retain the goal of ultimate and complete expulsion of the enemy from the territory of our own bodies. To "give up hope" for cure means becoming a "quitter."

Hope must never die, and heroism will be rewarded. Those presumptions shape our attitudes, dictate our decisions and are meant to sustain us through whatever tortures and treatments modern medical technology may dictate.

The problem with this paradigm, of course, is that death is certain. So, if to die is to "lose," then every human being, no matter how courageous, persistent, loving or eager to live, is a "loser" who "gave up." That can't be right.

I'm reminded of one young man with advanced testicular cancer who called our office for support in planning a peaceful death. At the time, Lance Armstrong's cancer survival and superhuman physical performance in the Tour de France filled the pages of popular magazines.

"I'm so tired of hearing about how Lance Armstrong 'beat' his cancer," he said. "Well, I'm not Lance Armstrong. It's clear I won't beat this."

Marjorie Williams, writing about her liver cancer in her posthumous 2006 book *The Woman at the Washington Zoo*, observed, "You'd be amazed how many people need to believe that only losers die of cancer."

These comments confirm my belief that when we cast overcoming an illness as a test of character, of strength or of will—even when overwhelming odds are against recovery—we send a message that stopping futile and torturous treatments is cowardly. If they remain gravely ill, patients often feel they have failed and let their loved ones down. People report feeling not just devastation, but shame when treatments are unsuccessful.

Unfortunately, Death Doesn't Care About Courage

Although we desperately need a new paradigm, the story of heroic battle repeatedly proves irresistible. Battling on and never quitting are such compelling ideals that lawmakers use them to political advantage and to justify excessive legal limitations on end-of-life choices.

In 2014, a 29-year-old woman named Brittany Maynard prompted much public dialogue when she moved from California to Oregon in order to gain access to medical aid in dying. When diagnosed with an aggressive brain tumor, Brittany asked about her prognosis and the symptoms she would experience before death. She decided she would like to have the option to escape the worst of those symptoms, if possible. So she moved her family, her furniture and her dogs to Portland, Oregon.

She continued treatment, but also qualified for medical aid in dying, authorized in Oregon but not in California at that time. Then she told her story to the nation, with the hope of preventing others from having to uproot themselves in order to obtain the peace of mind she had achieved. (Read the full inspiring story of Brittany in Chapter 10: People Taking Control.)

In 2014, another young person—32-year-old New Yorker James "JJ" Hanson—also rose to prominence in the ongoing national dialogue about medical aid in dying. Hanson had a glioblastoma, the same kind of brain tumor as Brittany Maynard. The difference between Brittany and JJ was that his tumor responded well to treatment and he enjoyed a period of remission, whereas surgery had sent Brittany's cancer into overdrive, on a relentless and invasive path of destruction.

Hanson lived three and a half years with his cancer. During this time, opponents of aid in dying rallied behind his inspiring commitment and perseverance. They positioned his "fight" as the courageous alternative to Brittany's "giving up." Hanson, a Marine veteran, adopted the tagline "Can't Hurt Steel," and his testimony to the press and legislators was that he would never back away from hope for a cure and a long life. His wife had a second child during this period, and he underwent many new and experimental treatments.

Brittany Maynard and JJ Hanson were the point/counterpoint in the medical aid-in-dying debate in Albany and other state capitols for several years. Brittany had already died, but her husband,

Dan Diaz, continued to testify about her illness, the treatment failures and her determined pursuit of a death on her own terms.

In the fall of 2017, Hanson ran out of treatment options. His cancer advancing, he left New York's Memorial Sloan Kettering Medical Center and entered hospice care in the home of his parents. He died December 30, 2017.

If any useful lesson can come from the twin telling of Brittany and JJ's stories, it is this: Cancer takes the courageous, the best and brightest stars in the human constellation just as surely as it takes anyone else. Courage and determination are ultimately no match for an aggressive, invasive cancer destined to kill. The fantasy of overcoming cancer, or any terminal illness, with sheer willpower is just a cruel delusion.

The idea that cancer kills only quitters may comfort us and insulate us from fear. But the comfort and insulation come at a price. We inadvertently denigrate those who might have fought the good fight but are now ready for gentle resignation. We press people who suspect the end is near to ignore their intuitive understanding and fight on. We steal the time they would otherwise have to close their lives and say goodbye. We rob them of the dignity of consciously and nobly taking their place in the great, sacred cycle and mystery of life.

The Costs of the Endless Fight

Is there a way to breach the false dichotomies of courage versus cowardice, of holding hope versus giving up?

In 2013, journalist Amanda Bennett delivered a TED talk based on her book *The Cost of Hope*. She told the story of a remarkable life with her husband, Terence, and their journey with kidney cancer. Her plea is for our society and our medical culture to write a new story about approaching death.

Amanda and Terence's story begins when she was in China as a young foreign correspondent. Meeting at a party, Terence dazzled her with his tales of studying Sino-Soviet relations as a Fulbright scholar. They talked for hours. She hung on his every word.

When she learned he actually represented the American Soybean Association, she confronted him. "I don't understand. Soybeans? You told me you were a Fulbright scholar."

"Well," he replied, "how long would you have talked to me if I told you I was in soybeans?"

Reader, she married him, and remained dazzled by him. Indeed, he was a dazzling man—fluent in six languages, proficient on fifteen musical instruments, a licensed pilot and a scholar of Chinese history. They had children, traveled the world and continued to be very much in love.

"It seemed like there was nothing that we couldn't do," Amanda said in her TED talk, "so when we found the cancer … we believed that, if we were smart enough and strong enough and brave enough, and we worked hard enough, we could keep him from dying ever."

She then described the next seven "exhilarating, glorious" years of battle against cancer, battles they kept winning. There were reprieves following setbacks: surgery, recurrence, a treatment that made Terence so sick he had to abandon it, internet research, more treatments, new ones, exotic ones and experimental ones. Throughout, they never believed this cancer would kill him. They remained confident new treatments would preserve his life. But eventually, the dark night came when a resident doctor in the ICU where Terence now was came to tell Amanda that Terence would die, perhaps before morning. He was 67.

Even in the face of this news, Amanda thought: *There's another drug out there. It's newer. It's more powerful … Perhaps there's still hope ahead.* So again, she asked the doctor to keep her husband alive if he could.

Amanda Bennett's book details the couple's earlier victories over kidney cancer, and their ordeal. Their hope had a literal cost, of course, which amounted to $618,616. This sum represents, among other things, pills that carried a price tag of $200 each, $735 for each injection of Interleukin-2 (an agent that uses the body's natural immune system to fight cancer) and $27,360 for each dose of Avastin (a chemotherapy drug that inhibits growth of a tumor's blood supply). The couple was among those in America lucky enough to be fully insured and not forced to bear the brunt of that price tag.

But there were also the less tangible costs of clinging to unending hope: the costs to them in comfort, quality of life, emotional reckoning and psychological readiness, especially for younger family members.

"People did mention hospice, but I wouldn't listen," says Bennett. "Hospice was for people who were dying, and Terence wasn't dying." In an article for *Bloomberg Businessweek*, she later reflected, "Looking back, memories of my zeal to treat are tinged with sadness. Should I have given up earlier? Would earlier hospice care have been kinder? I hadn't believed Terence was going to die so I had never confronted any of those dilemmas. And I never let us have the chance to say goodbye."

Soon after the resident doctor's pronouncement, Terence entered a coma. He never left the hospital again, and spent only four days under hospice care. He remained in the same hospital bed. The doctors simply took away the monitors and machines, and different staff members—hospice nurses, chaplains and counselors—replaced the hospitalists and oncologists.

"We pushed the fight right over the edge," Bennett says. The final cost of their inexhaustible hope was the tender goodbyes left unsaid and the conscious reconciliation with being mortal that they did not achieve.

A Hero's Farewell

Amanda Bennett rejects any suggestion that "hope" is just a nice word for denial. She sees hope, even irrational hope, as a desirable and necessary trait that protects us and keeps us engaged in life. Comparing humans to software, she says hope is "... not a bug, but a feature" of being human.

Rather than abandoning hope, she suggests, we need to re-write the end-of-life story. The new version needs to be one of valor, as inspiring as any tale of feats of courage on a battlefield. The new story need not be about losing hope or giving up; it can still be a story of brave soldiering and valiant victories. But this version ends with a gradual recognition that bravery can no longer carry the day, and that the time has finally come for graceful retreat.

A single heroic act is the turning point in this story. That act is the conscious recognition that a life has been completed and the time has come to die. This story acknowledges that no treatment has ever made a person immortal, and death eventually comes to us all. This story, Bennett suggests, could give us a "noble path to dying," a "heroic narrative for letting go."

I share Bennett's conviction that humans are compelled to cherish hope and keep it alive until the moment of their deaths. But I also believe what we hope *for* can, and must, change. Ultimately, the final hope may be that we be allowed to bid the world a hero's farewell. To do this, we must be alert enough and informed enough to discern the perfect timing for surrender and retreat. We must understand what our doctors understand about the course of disease and the futility of treatment. Only then can we make the noble decision to accept the fate we share with all living creatures and exit this life with grace and dignity.

Brave New Stories

In her TED Talk, Amanda Bennett shares lines from "The God Abandons Antony," a poem about Marc Antony's defeat and retreat from Alexandria, Egypt, written by the Greek poet Constantine P. Cavafy. I'm more familiar with the derivative 2001 Leonard Cohen song "Alexandra Leaving," about the sad acceptance of a love ending. Both the poem and the song instruct one who faces a great loss to bear it without regret or self-pity. "Go firmly to the window," Cavafy instructs Marc Antony. Go, he says, "as one long prepared, and graced with courage, say goodbye to her"—the city of Alexandria Antony was about to leave behind. Above all, Cavafy advises, don't pretend you haven't noticed the impending doom and don't degrade yourself with empty delusion. In Cohen's song version, he also counsels, "Do not stoop to strategies like this."

This is how a hero leaves the field of battle—proudly, consciously and with a sad, calm resolve.

The American sportscaster, Stuart Scott, offered just such a brave new story in the face of his own terminal cancer, in 2014. "When you die, that does not mean that you lose to cancer," he said, at an awards ceremony six months before his death. "You beat cancer by how you live, why you live and the manner in which you live."

I would add that this also means you beat cancer in the way you live your death. To many, dying is not the greatest defeat. Or, in the words of my dear friend and mentor Rev. Dr. Paul Smith, "Dying is not the worst thing that can happen to you." The worst thing, the greatest defeat, is when cancer or any other disease robs us, in the process of dying, of everything it means to be human. This includes all experiences of the mind and body: thinking, loving, praying and filling our hearts and the hearts of those around us with gratitude for the miracles of life and beauty. Escaping the continuation of "mere existence" when all other gifts of human life are gone—that is the final victory to be won.

What We Hope for Can Change as Terminal Illness Progresses

Our hopes during an experience with terminal illness, whether it be our own or that of a loved one, can change as the disease progresses and death is nearer. Here is an example of progression of hope in a terminal-illness experience, from diagnosis through to the final days of life.

- Hope the diagnosis is wrong. There's been some sort of error.
- Hope for a total cure. Robust health and expectation of long life will return.
- Hope for slowing progression of the disease, that life may be extended.
- Hope that pain and other symptoms don't cause unbearable suffering.
- Hope that dying leaves those who remain with peaceful memories of love and life completion.
- "Healed" hope. Hope that transcends any specific "wish." Hope in the wholeness of participation in the glory and mysteries of life and death.

6

Hospice: The Healing Option

W ould earlier hospice care have been kinder?" Amanda Bennett asks in the article she wrote for *Bloomberg* about her husband Terence's battle to the end, and the answer is, in a word, "Yes."

Hospice is the best setting for a hero's retreat and a hero's farewell. I have heard many individuals and their families describe the tranquility that descended upon them as soon as hospice workers arrived in the home, with their sweet candor about the journey ahead and their swift attention to the physical comfort and emotional peace of the dying person. I have felt that tranquility myself. After the frenetic strain of a futile fight, it feels like a miracle. Every hero deserves a supportive environment, a resting place from which to, as songwriter Leonard Cohen wrote, "go firmly to the window, drink it in." Hospice provides the vantage point from which one can step into the honor of living and dying in grace.

To me, it seems like the most natural thing, to want to die at home surrounded by beloved people and things. But sadly, American media often treats this choice as an aberration.

Dying at Home Still Grabs Headlines

Around the same time in 2018 that headlines were incorrectly depicting Senator John McCain in a *mano a mano* battle with brain cancer, other headlines described former first lady Barbara Bush and her suddenly public last days.

Mrs. Bush had suffered shortness of breath for months, caused by congestive heart failure and chronic obstructive pulmonary disease (COPD). She repeatedly received hospital treatment, with diminishing returns. Finally, the 92-year-old made a conscious decision to return home for good, with a new focus on "comfort care." Her decision was pointedly made public on April 16, National Healthcare Decisions Day.

The decision by the former first lady to hop off the medical conveyor belt and face her terminal illness with new goals for care was blown up by the press, becoming a media storm. Their overly dramatic and downbeat stories used phrases like "declines medical treatment" and "giving up" and reported that Bush's decision had sparked a national debate on what it means to "stop fighting" a terminal illness. This negative reporting was due in part to the family's confusing public statement, which said that Barbara had decided "not to seek additional medical treatment and will focus on comfort care." Statements like this confuse people, because they suggest that comfort care is not "treatment."

As Haider Warraich, cardiac doctor, author of *Modern Death*, and a Compassion & Choices board member, pointed out in a widely circulated *Kaiser Health News* interview at the time, "One of the common myths about palliative care is that they [patients] are being denied medical help." Instead, he explained, "comfort care" usually means opting not to use a breathing machine or CPR, but patients will continue to receive medical treatment, such as morphine, to ease shortness of breath, and diuretics to remove excess fluid from their lungs. Doctors and specialists remain very much engaged with their patients as they deliver comfort care to them.

Did Barbara Bush make the right decision for herself? Readers who continued to follow her story after the family's statement learned that Barbara's last days at home were probably exactly as she had hoped. Just prior to her death, the Bushes' longtime friend Ambassador C. Boyden Gray said Barbara was in good spirits, answering phone calls and writing emails. Another source close to the Bush family told CBS News reporter Jenna Gibson that Barbara "was alert and was having conversations last night. She was also having a bourbon." Comfort care indeed!

I agree with Dr. Warraich that "by bringing this into the sphere of discussion, we can start thinking about comfort and palliation long before we are in the clutches of death." But I can't help but find ridiculous the furor around a 92-year-old woman deciding to die at home surrounded by her loved ones, rather than in a hospital, attached to a breathing machine. Barbara Bush's timing of her death was her own call to make, but I do hope she gained much satisfaction and joy from the bourbon, and the love, in her home.

The Pull of Familiar Surroundings

Most hospice care takes place in the home, and that is where the majority of people say they would choose to die. People want to be among the things that exemplify their life at its peak of experience and meaning. When Jacqueline Kennedy Onassis received the news from doctors at the New York Hospital that no further treatment would help her, she retreated to her home on 5th Avenue. It was her wish to die in the company of the art and the books that had enriched and sustained her. Our homes house the symbols of our story: loved ones, memories, accomplishments, ecstasies and tragedies, too. Dying in our story means, whenever possible, dying at home.

If it is difficult for an adult who is dying to persuade doctors and loved ones to let them die naturally at home, for a child it is practically impossible. Yet even a child can feel the pull of familiar surroundings, and will talk about this, if allowed.

A New York pediatrician tells of a six-year-old boy, a kindergarten classmate of her own son, hospitalized for a neuroblastoma. She became close to the mother and visited the boy regularly in the hospital during many of his 39 cycles of chemotherapy and 27 surgeries.

She describes one of these visits, when he was growing weaker and no options to prolong his life remained:

"He was very weak. We spent some time drawing together, and he told me he was sick of the hospital. Often, he had told me stories of angels hanging out outside. But on this day, he looked into my eyes and said, 'Talk to my mom. She will listen to you. You need to tell her I want to die at home, not here. I want my friends to visit. I want to hear my sister play piano. And I would like to just enjoy whatever time is left. I hate the smells and rules of the hospital. Will you do that? Will you speak with my mom, please?'" This wise and articulate little boy, after suffering so much painful treatment, bravely spoke of what mattered most to him in the final phase of his life. At the age of six, he displayed more serenity and courage in the face of death than countless adults can summon. His request was heard—he died at home.

This private story echoes a very public one, chronicled by CNN in 2015. Julianna Snow was a four-year-old with a rare and incurable illness that left her muscles too feeble to support her standing or moving and her respiratory muscles too weak to clear secretions in her lungs. Hers was a constant struggle to breathe and avoid a lethal pneumonia.

Her parents took care of her at home. Especially torturous was the procedure in which respiratory therapists pushed a suction catheter up Julianna's nose and down into her trachea, causing her to gag and cough violently. Given the choice, Julianna would choose her father over respiratory therapists to pass the tube and suction out the mucus. Both father and child suffered mightily during these procedures, occurring *every four hours, around the clock*. Julianna had to be restrained during these treatments and she dreaded them.

Her mother, Michelle Moon, set off a storm of controversy when she blogged about the family's decision to respect the child's wishes during the next medical emergency. Her parents had asked Julianna where she would rather go when she experienced her next infection: the hospital or heaven. Julianna chose heaven.

The blog reported their conversation.

Michelle: "Julianna, if you get sick again, do you want to go to the hospital again or stay home?"

Julianna: "Not the hospital."

Michelle: "Even if that means that you will go to heaven if you stay home?"

Julianna: "Yes."

Michelle: "And you know that mommy and daddy won't come with you right away? You'll go by yourself first."

Julianna: "Don't worry. God will take care of me."

Michelle: "And if you go to the hospital, it may help you get better and let you come home again and spend more time with us. I need to make sure you understand that. The hospital may let you have more time with mommy and daddy."

Julianna: "I understand."

At home again, Julianna was completely dependent on a mask hooked up to a machine for breathing assistance. Lying in her bed, in a room decorated as a princess fantasy, Julianna chose a different princess dress to wear each day. She retained total clarity regarding her conviction that nothing was worth the torture of another hospital stay and more suctioning treatments.

Once Julianna was home for good, with comfort as the only goal, Michelle described life in hospice as stable and wonderful. The benefits included immediate access to medical advice, regular visits from an aide, meetings with a bereavement counselor and four hours each week with a "hospice angel" who entertained Julianna.

Michelle said, "Now my focus is different. I am no longer consumed by doing everything I can to work against Julianna's disease. It is easier to give her my undivided attention and just enjoy her. I think Julianna senses this and it has helped her thrive."

The point of these stories is that it is indeed possible to "heal" or "thrive," in a larger sense, even when a person will not "recover." Healing carries a broader and deeper meaning than "curing." "Thriving" can be a condition of the spirit, if not the body. It's difficult, but important, to attune ourselves to those things that may promote "healing," or "thriving," even while dying. Often, being at home is crucial for this to occur.

What Exactly Is Hospice?

A shift in focus, from cure to comfort, is the defining heroic moment in our new story of dying of terminal illness. Patients can stop squandering precious time and energy enduring torturous treatments if this shift occurs. When hope for a cure has passed, a patient-directed approach and the practice of hospice care help patients and their loved ones replace hope for a cure with the hope for healing.

I consider hospice to be the gold standard of end-of life care. I say this because of its integration in urban and rural communities across the nation, for its history and experience in the interdisciplinary team model and for its concentration on spiritual and emotional well-being, long before palliative care was recognized as a medical specialty.

Hospice is both a type and a philosophy of care that focuses on supporting and comforting a gravely ill individual. The concept evolved in Europe, beginning in the 11th century, as a place of rest for pilgrims and travelers. It changed over time into a place where the sick, wounded or dying received hospitality and care. A woman named Cicely Saunders started the first modern hospice in 1967 in Great Britain. In America today, hospice is largely understood according to its Medicare definition: a holistic model of treatment reserved for individuals who are within six months of death and who have exhausted treatments aimed at curing the illness or prolonging life.

Hospice is not a place, like a hospital, nor one organization. Rather, as stated above, it is a concept of care that focuses on comfort for the patient rather than cure for the illness. This model of care is built around managing physical symptoms, such as pain, anxiety and shortness of breath, and trying to make the most of the present moment, rather than dwelling on the uncertainties of the future. Hospice aims to help people enjoy their last season of life. It also aims to support patients, and their friends and family, emotionally, socially and spiritually.

Most communities today have several hospice organizations operating nearby. As with any medical services, the quality of hospices can vary greatly. Asking careful questions can ensure that you select the hospice that best meets your needs (see box).

I like to think that hospice holds a place for the firm walk to the window that I mentioned in the previous chapter, offering a space for the long drinking in of all the sweet joy and sacred sorrow of a full and conscious life. Hospice's effectiveness in helping people complete their lives while arriving at a place of healing rests on its structure and philosophy.

A key benefit of hospice is that it enables and increases the probability of a person dying at home. In the next section, I explain many other benefits of the hospice approach and its relationship to hospitals and the palliative care specialty that has arisen in the past 20 years, approximately. Most especially, it seems to me, hospice enables the hero's ending that we might seek.

The Benefits of Hospice

Hospice is holistic. Hospice care extends beyond the body. It focuses on the emotional and spiritual well-being of patients, as well as their physical comfort. A hospice team includes physicians, nurses, clergy, dieticians, home health aides, counselors, social workers, and volunteers, offering a range of therapeutic services. Because hospice care most often takes place in the home, patients retain access to whatever books, music, poetry and prayers have sustained and nurtured their spirit throughout life. Familiar smells, including the smell of favorite foods cooking, evoke the joy and fullness of life.

Hospice aids the family. Beyond providing assistance during the final phase of a patient's life, hospice offers grief counseling and may even assist with some of the responsibilities facing the family after a loved one has passed away.

Hospice offers dignity and tranquility. Anyone who has spent time in a hospital, even for an event as commonplace as giving birth, knows how challenging it can be to have peace and privacy. Medical personnel enter your room at will at all hours of the day and night. Monitors and other machines flash and beep. Meals arrive according to the hospital's schedule. Patients are prodded and poked and may overhear impersonal teaching discussions of which they are the subject. With a transfer to hospice at home, patients are restored to their own sphere of autonomy, with few of the disturbances and indignities of a hospital setting.

Hospice may extend your life. Ironically, some people who have exhausted treatments aimed at curing illness or prolonging life enroll in hospice for their final days, and then go on to live longer than expected (and in a nicer fashion than in the hospital). We cannot know exactly the reasons for this, but we do know that groups of cancer and heart disease patients enrolled in hospice or receiving palliative care services live longer, on average, than patients who receive only treatments to fight their disease and none to ensure their comfort.

Hospice relieves financial anxieties by preventing costly hospitalizations at the very end. Patients can be acutely aware that hospital bills are often staggering. Indeed, medical costs are a major cause of bankruptcy in the United States. However, most managed care plans, insurance policies and health maintenance organizations (HMOs) cover hospice care in full, and anyone on Medicare pays little or nothing for its services.

In November 2014, the *Journal of the American Medical Association* published a study on the end-of-life care of more than 36,000 patients, conducted by Dr. Ziad Obermeyer, a health policy specialist at Harvard Medical School. Dr. Obermeyer and his colleagues compared two groups of older Americans with metastatic cancer. One group was enrolled in hospice and the other group was not. The researchers tracked the patients until they died.

Medicare records revealed the patients enrolled in hospice had far fewer hospitalizations and fewer than half as many visits to the ICU, compared to those who were not enrolled in hospice. They were subjected to 50 percent fewer invasive procedures and they were five times less likely to die in an institutional setting. Finally, the cost of end-of-life care was almost $9,000 less per patient for those in hospice. Dr. Obermeyer estimates these savings, if extended nationwide, could amount to billions of dollars.

The same is true for visits to the emergency room. In 2012,

Health Affairs published a study examining the emergency department visits of patients aged 65 or older. Alexander Smith, a geriatrician at the University of California San Francisco (UCSF), found that nearly half of the 4,000 patients in the study visited the emergency department during the final month of life, while 75 percent did so during the last six months of life. Moreover, 77 percent of those visits resulted in a hospital admission, and 68 percent of these hospitalized patients never returned home. Conversely, patients who had enrolled in hospice at least one month before death were rarely transported to an emergency department during their final month of life.

Hospice financial incentives align with patient well-being. Hospices receive payment from Medicare and other insurers at a set rate per day. The rate varies by intensity of service, but is not affected by specific treatments. To receive any payments at all, hospices must meet strict standards for the quality and scope of services provided. Thus, hospices have an incentive to deliver comprehensive care as efficiently as possible.

Hospitals generally receive payment according to how many procedures and services they provide. The more procedures, and the more intense the treatments and care, the higher the payment they receive. I'm not saying hospitals operate on greed, but we would be foolish to think they are immune to the influence of financial incentives, which may lead to more unnecessary or overly-intensive treatments than is always desirable.

Policy leaders have long understood the perverse problem caused by the fee-for-service hospital payment structure. In fact, the Medicare Access and CHIP Reauthorization Act of 2015 attempts to address this problem by implementing an alternative payment model, which moves hospitals away from fee-for-service structures which can encourage overtreatment. However, it will take years to fully implement this policy and it impacts only Medicare reimbursements. We are still a long way away from having a hospital payment structure that does not reward overtreatment.

Meanwhile, claims by extremists that hospices are working to "kill" patients for financial gain are ignorant and irrational. An example of that irrational thinking showed up in a *60 Minutes II* segment which aired on June 22, 1999. It featured a case involving a woman who died in hospice and was found to have high blood levels of morphine. Dr. Ronald Reeves, Coroner of Volusia County, Florida, ruled the death a homicide. He also asserted that hospice personnel often administer morphine specifically to cause the death of their patients. The specter that financial gain could be a contributing motive often accompanies such claims.

The reality, however, is that payments to both hospitals and hospices *cease* when a patient dies. Both, then, have zero incentive to enable the premature death of a patient.

Choosing a Good Hospice Program

Your doctors or the Medicare.gov website can direct you to prospective hospice programs in your area. When you first contact these programs, find out the following:

- Is the hospice provider certified and licensed by the state or federal government?
- Does the hospice provider train caregivers to care for you at home?
- How will your doctor work with the doctor from the hospice provider?
- How many patients are assigned to each member of the hospice care staff?
- Will the hospice staff meet regularly with you and your family to discuss care?
- How does the hospice staff respond to after-hours emergencies?
- What measures are in place to ensure the high quality of hospice care?
- What services do hospice volunteers offer? Are they trained?
- In jurisdictions where medical aid in dying is authorized, does the hospice support patients who wish to request this option?

See also "How to Interview a Hospice" at CompassionAndChoices. org/endoflifeplanning.

The All-Important Transfer from
Hospitalization to Hospice

In the mid-1980s, the number of deaths occurring in hospital settings was the highest in the 20th century, accounting for 54 to 60 percent of all deaths recorded. Medicare set up its payment system for hospice in 1982, largely in response to a growing perception of hospitals' poor-quality care for terminally ill patients. Hospital culture, with a compelling ethic to delay death regardless of the cost in technology, pain and suffering, had become inhumane in the opinion of many dying patients.

Since that time, the location of death has shifted away from hospitals. Hospital deaths accounted for only 19.8 percent of all deaths in 2015. This proportion is considered highly desirable, because it aligns with measurable indicators of high-quality healthcare and reflects what people say they want.

Concurrently, utilization of hospice has risen sharply in recent years, but a mere rise in the percentage of people who die while in hospice care is misleading. One telling indicator of little progress is that despite the increase in use of hospice care, admissions to the ICU during the last 30 days of life are rising. Yes, more people are dying while in hospice care than ever, but this doesn't necessarily reflect better patient experiences, because transfer to hospice often comes so very late in the patient's downward course. Hospitals continue to treat dying patients with great intensity—admitting them to intensive care units, subjecting them to painful interventions and discharging them to hospice mere hours or days before death. We saw an example of this in the previous chapter, with the case of the comatose Terence Bennett.

Why do hospitals bother to transfer patients to hospice at all? Hospitals want to transfer patients to hospice because these patients would otherwise die in the hospital. For obvious marketing reasons, no hospital wants its in-hospital death rate to exceed the national average or that of its local competitors.

Patients may get recorded as dying under hospice care, but the experience is more akin to a hospital death, because inhumane technology prevailed almost to the very end. These barely conscious patients, transferred so late to hospice, sadly derive little benefit from hospice's psycho-spiritual supports.

My summary of the situation is that hospitalization is appropriate so long as the benefit of intensive treatment outweighs its burdens. Hospice does its best work when patients have time to rest in physical comfort and engage in the psycho-spiritual work of healing into dying. So, the timing of the transition from hospital to hospice is crucial, but often way off the mark, happening much too late in the dying process. This is a worrisome trend and an abuse of hospice that warrants monitoring.

A Few Words About the Palliative Care Specialty

While palliative care is a component of hospice care, palliative care apart from the hospice model is mostly hospital-based. The palliative care specialty is concentrated in large institutions and teaching hospitals across the nation, and it is a relative newcomer (within the last 20 years) on the scene of end-of-life care.

As defined by the Center to Advance Palliative Care's website:

Palliative care, and the medical sub-specialty of palliative medicine, is medical care for people living with serious illness. It focuses on providing relief from the symptoms and stress of a serious illness. The goal is to improve quality of life for both the patient and the family.

Palliative care is provided by a team of palliative care doctors, nurses, social workers and others who work together with a patient's other doctors to provide an extra layer of support. It is appropriate at any age and at any stage in a serious illness and can be provided along with curative treatment.

Palliative care serves a very importance niche, as it provides patients who are not yet terminal with much needed comfort and services and allows them to begin thinking about the quality of their life. However, I have been disappointed by the insistence of some leaders in the palliative care community that palliative care doctors should avoid words like *death, dying, end-of-life* or *terminal.*

As an example, one of the most prominent and respected leaders in the field of palliative care said in an interview, "It's not our job as health professionals to be convincing people that it's OK to die, and that death is natural and death is good. It flies in the face of millions of years of human evolution. It's not OK to die." She went on to say, "Quite naturally, all living things try to avoid death, and are afraid of death. And by focusing on that inevitable event, you're not living in the present. You're letting your life be defined by the fear of death."

My experience is quite different. What I have found is that often people are able to live life to the fullest precisely *because* they have accepted the inevitability of death. Hiding from the only certain thing in life—death—does not decrease the likelihood that it will take place. Understanding death does allow you to make choices that maximize your quality of life.

Patients receiving palliative care with no notification from a medical professional that they are approaching death are robbed of the opportunity to say goodbye to their loved ones and to put priorities in place for the final months of their life.

Given their aversion to discussing death or hospice, some leaders in the palliative care community are also, by extension, opposed to medical aid in dying. If the goal of palliative care is to "help patients and families understand the nature of their illness and make timely, informed decisions about their care," I wonder how this can be achieved without a forthright discussion that the disease is beyond cure and life is drawing to a close? Medical professionals who refuse to acknowledge death are failing to address a critical part of a person's disease, and they are failing to fully support the caregivers who are left behind. As a result, they are less valuable partners for those ready to be truly present in their deaths—present for the changes in mind and spirit that psychiatrist and author Elisabeth Kübler-Ross outlined in her description of dying, which she called "the final stage of growth." (In Chapters 2, 3 and 7, particularly, we provide the questions to ask if readers sense a doctor is not being candid with them or their loved one.)

I will note that I have had the pleasure of working with many wonderful palliative care doctors who are skilled at moving a patient along the continuum care spectrum, from serious illness to terminal disease, engaging in forthright conversations every step of the way. When the palliative care leadership and community embrace and recognize what these doctors are practicing, we as a country will be in a position to benefit from the full promise of palliative care.

The Need for Palliative Care: Two Illustrative Tales

It's easy to take for granted the benefits that modern-day palliative care confers on those at the end of life. I share with you the following two stories, which demonstrate the enormous difference advances in palliative care can make.

The very worst death I ever witnessed was that of a man hospitalized with pulmonary fibrosis. He sat bolt upright in bed, gasping, straining and panting in misery because his lungs were unable to extract enough oxygen from the 100 percent concentration delivered to the small tented enclosure around his head. Sweat ran down his face, and his body was close to total exhaustion with the enormous effort he sustained, hour after hour. The medical staff did little except wait for him to tire and collapse. No one would give him morphine, which would have vastly lessened his misery, as doing so would have also hastened his death, by dulling the desperate drive or sensation of needing to breathe.

A more kind and humane intervention would have been to acknowledge to this man that his super-human efforts to breathe were brave and heroic. But no hero wins every battle, and it is also heroic to summon the courage to leave the field while it is still possible to bequeath sweet and decent memories to those who will live with the images of this day. A doctor could have shared this truth and offered medication to ease the sense of suffocation. Then it would have been possible for his distraught wife to witness her husband taking his last few breaths without terror in his eyes. This would have been the kinder course of action, but no one wanted to accept the responsibility of "causing" his death by giving him morphine. So, the man struggled on, his wife unable to bear being at his side, and he died after three days of pure torture.

Contrast that with the following story of the skillful use of morphine and sedatives to enable one man's heroic journey to the completion of this life and the experience of a gentle, loving death.

In 1992, before a certified palliative care medical specialty was in existence, Drs. Miles J. Edwards and Susan W. Tolle of Oregon Health and Sciences University described an exemplary palliative treatment in their article in *Annals of Internal Medicine*. The article was a poignant account of their soul searching in response to a patient's request to discontinue the ventilator that kept him alive. These two physicians were called upon to allow a patient to live his "new heroism" into death, as they removed the ventilator and provided medication to sedate him and suppress the respiratory drive. This was good medicine, and their candor was good ethics.

The patient, Mr. Larson, was in late middle age when he developed post-polio syndrome. Rapidly progressive weakness and shortness of breath required hospitalization, a tracheostomy and continuous mechanical ventilation. All consultants agreed he would never again breathe independent of a ventilator. After days of contemplation, Mr. Larson asked to discontinue it. He was fully aware he would die once this was accomplished. He underwent a psychiatric evaluation and was deemed competent to make decisions. There was some initial resistance from his three adult children, but after their own dialogue and reflection they agreed to support his decision. After all, who would again inflict involuntary immobilization and confinement on a polio victim who had earlier managed to escape the imprisonment of an iron lung and live free?

"Then came the particularly difficult question: how would this be done with compassion and with a minimum of suffering?" the physicians recalled in their article. They acknowledged that, "Any use of sedative or narcotic analgesic medication to relieve the unwanted sensation [of suffocation] would also reduce respiratory

When a Loved One Enters Hospice at Home

Despite hospice's enormous benefits, it is wise to understand potential difficulties and anticipate them. It's certainly easier for all involved if a person enters hospice care sooner rather than later. But whether you have the time to research and prepare for hospice at home or events suddenly take a turn and your loved one is abruptly enrolled into a home hospice program, here are some things to keep in mind.

Understand what home hospice does and doesn't do.
At the intake session with hospice, make sure that all questions are aired, both by the patient and, if necessary, privately between caretakers and the hospice coordinator. Learn the scope and limitations of what hospice can daily do for you. Ask about access to a doctor and find out the schedule of when nurses will come to the house, and what will happen during those visits.

If the nurse hands you a "comfort box," request to carefully go over the contents of the box together and discuss when and how the contents are to be used.
Home hospice workers are not allowed to dispense medications like morphine and anti-anxiety drugs, so you will need some instruction. Take notes.

As you set up hospice at home, get the equipment and services you need.
Will the hospice service provide an electric hospital bed, a rolling table, a walker, a commode? How about a bathing basin, sponges, adult diapers and sippy cups? Do you have the necessary pillows (all sizes), cooling patches, sheets, blankets and towels?

Two quality-of-life services to request from the hospice on behalf of the patient are professional bathing and massage with therapeutic oils, if available. And if those services are available but for some reason aren't provided, request again.

drive; the two are inseparable."

The doctors were very mindful of their patient's humanity. They did not undertake this action lightly. When the time came to honor his request, they asked him to confirm that his wishes had not

---

While you may have many people helping out, appoint one decision person from the start.
Things change rapidly as the end of life approaches, and continuity of care can be a big issue in home hospice, with a rotating group of service providers and family members showing up at different times. One designated family member or friend should have the overview of the home hospice situation and be given the latitude to set the ground rules and delegate whatever, to whomever, as needed.

Frontload "the good moments."
Hospice is about quality time. Identify early what makes a difference to your loved one and make that a priority. Does she love nature? Make sure there's access to a sunny window or a nice plant in the room. Are there favorite music or movies that he loves? Play them now. Is there a food she's craving? Ask every day because it may change. Are there children or other special people that you know your loved one should see? Don't wait for "a good time" to invite them—the sooner they come the better.

If you decide you need or want 24/7 care at home, you will probably need to hire it privately.
In-home aides can be expensive but may be necessary if the person in hospice needs constant supervision due to terminal agitation or a rapidly changing condition. No matter how solicitous, family caregivers need to get sleep and coordinate events beyond the hospice room, and hiring an aide to watch over the patient and generally help out may be crucial. Get names of aide services and interview them at the beginning of the hospice process so that they are just a phone call away if needed.

Understand that you are saying goodbye to your loved one, not trying to nurse him or her back to health.
Look to maximize the quiet, loving moments of shared smiles and stories, and minimize the unwanted, invasive medical moments, which may keep intruding even at the very end.

changed, and they described what he might experience during the process. They explained that they could not know precisely how much medication would relieve his feeling of air hunger upon coming off the ventilator. If he began to struggle, they sought his permission to reconnect him to the apparatus briefly, while they calmly administered more medication. They also promised him morphine to ensure his comfort if he did not die as soon as expected.

The procedure went smoothly. At the one brief point when the patient became slightly breathless, they increased the dose of drugs. After this, "Mr. Larson seemed comfortable, breathing shallowly at a rate of 28 [breaths]/minute. He exchanged smiles with his daughter, who stood holding his hand across the bed. He appeared reasonably comfortable and relaxed." After about 30 minutes, the patient slipped gradually into a coma.

After another 15 minutes, his breathing became irregular and eventually it ceased. He was no longer attached to any monitors, which the doctors believed lessened the family's stress during the patient's final moments. His heartbeat became irregular and intermittent. "We took turns listening and waited until we were certain that he had died," the doctors reported. "Fifty-three minutes after he was disconnected from the vent, we pronounced him dead." The doctors then received grateful hugs from the family and thanks from the health care team. For its honesty, brevity, gentleness and mercy on all involved, I consider this a heroic death indeed.

An Integrated Healing

For the reasons above, I recommend investigating the availability of hospice when the hope for a cure has passed, so that it can be replaced by the hope for healing. What is this "healing" that enables one to find a new hero's story in dying? Author Stephen Levine says it is "the harmonizing of the disquieted, a balancing of energies to bring about peace where before there had been war ... the integration of body and mind into the heart."

For decades Stephen and Ondrea Levine directed Hanuman Foundation Dying Project. They counseled thousands of people confronting serious illness, grief or death. Stephen's books, including *Who Dies* and *Healing into Life and Death,* share the profound wisdom gained through these encounters and the meditative practices they found most helpful.

When they began their work, Stephen and Ondrea shared the common belief that healing was of the body. But they came to see it as a force operating on many levels of mind, body and spirit. Healing can occur even as disease continues to progress. Indeed, this is a common experience for those nearing death consciously. For the Levines, healing means the freedom to experience the "wholeness of death," and the fullness of the moment.

So, our new story of heroism is the turning from frantic searches for a cure to the calm opening of the heart and the freeing of the spirit. Levine writes of people achieving, at the end of life, a "painful grace," but also a "quiet completion" and "greater wellness." These people "were more healed, more whole at the moment in their dying than at any time in their life," he writes. "They had healed into death, their business finished, their future wide open."

We may make the story of our dying one of being ennobled by the conscious acceptance of our destiny. To live courageously is to savor each moment, to savor life even as it is transient. To die heroically is to savor it all, even the bright sadness of leaving.

7

The Secret of Slow Medicine

The term "slow medicine" doesn't sound like a cutting-edge medical breakthrough. No modern hospital is likely to use the phrase for bragging rights in its marketing materials. But in light of Chapter 3, which outlined the various pressures to overtreat, slowing down decisions about any test or treatment is important. It takes time to consider alternatives, weigh benefits and burdens and check in with your own values and priorities. Often a tragic cascade of pain and suffering can be traced back to one crucial step, taken without thinking through the consequences.

Another impetus to slow medicine down is the desire to align treatment with forces of nature and optimize the body's own remarkable capacity for healing. Each medical intervention carries a risk of harm. And more often than we would like to think, more harm than good comes from medical tests, hospitalization, medication and surgical procedures.

The term "iatrogenic disease" describes a disease caused by a medical intervention. Study after study confirms that medical error and iatrogenic illness account for at least 100,000 deaths per year, making this the third most common cause of death in the nation. Add to this statistic the many more people who just become sicker or disabled, or have a longer recovery time, due to the side effects or errors in treatment. Slow medicine seeks to reduce these extraordinary risks by allowing time to assess options, thus eliminating unnecessary and potentially risky tests, treatments and hospitalizations. Let's explore how it works.

I had a gardening accident several years ago. After an early morning of planting corn and cultivating beans, I strained to pull off my rubber gardening clogs. As I did so, I heard a soft pop and felt a zinging sensation along the top of my finger. The ligament holding the finger straight had snapped and the tip of my right middle digit hung limp, at a right angle. It didn't hurt, but the finger was decidedly out of commission.

I called my friend and colleague Charlie, a retired hand surgeon, to ask whether I should go straight from the garden to the nearest emergency room.

"I wouldn't," he replied. "A surgeon is more likely to make it worse than make it better. My advice is to stay away from emergency rooms and surgeons."

What to do, then?

"Splint it in a position with the tip tilting up and keep it there for eight weeks," he instructed. *"Don't let the fingertip drop*, or the healing process will be ruined. I'll send you special splints."

In a nutshell, this is slow medicine: helping the body heal itself and having the patience to wait until it does. I used a Popsicle stick to hold my finger still until Charlie's package arrived. Then I carefully positioned the splint, wrapped my finger, and kept it dry with a rubber finger cot. When eight weeks had passed, I peeked at the finger. It was still drooping slightly so I reapplied the splint and waited another 4 weeks. This time when I unveiled my finger—*voilà!*—it had healed completely.

Charlie's slow approach actually saved me a lot of time. It spared me the pain and trauma of hand surgery and the risk of a surgical error, wound infection or other calamity. And incidentally, it also saved me and my insurance carrier a bundle of money.

Slow medicine is a worthy course of action for injuries like mine, where the body can heal itself if we give it the time and support to do so. It is also often the best approach for frail bodies wracked by advanced illness. This is because it avoids the risk of incidental harm and a cascade of undesirable side effects that can further weaken a diseased body or bring greater disability.

When Patience and Humility Guide Your Care

The principles of slow medicine have special significance when illnesses like cancer or lung disease have taken their toll—when a patient's condition is severe and their body frail and weak. Dr. Myron Turbow, a medical consultant for Compassion & Choices who practiced for decades as an oncologist and hospice director, says he learned three essential tenets of good care during his career. "As an oncologist, I learned that some things can't be fixed," he told me. "No matter what you do, you can't fix them. Then as a hospice director, I learned some things *shouldn't* be fixed. For example, let's say a cancer patient comes in with a bowel obstruction. Do you send them to surgery for the bowel obstruction even though they're full of cancer and it would take weeks, even in the best of circumstances, to recover from that so-called 'simple surgery'? Because there is another option, which is to just keep a person with end-stage terminal cancer comfortable. Or let's say a very frail and elderly person with a terminal illness comes in with pneumonia. Well, the pneumonia we can fix! We can give antibiotics for that. But the question is: should we? Because they're going to die soon in some way, and pneumonia can be a much gentler way to go than they might experience otherwise."

The point Dr. Turbow makes is that a peaceful death from pneumonia can be far less traumatic than the intense agony of bowel obstruction or the torment of surgery and the recovery from it.

He sums up, "So, I learned there are things that can't be fixed. I learned there are things that shouldn't be fixed. And I learned the *power of presence*. There's a tremendous power in the simple willingness to remain fully present with a patient."

To anyone unfamiliar with our medical culture today, these tenets might sound self-evident. But anyone who knows our current healthcare system will recognize how rarely this kind of patience and humility guides patient care. Dr. Turbow readily acknowledges that our present-day medical culture has a built-in resistance to restraint.

"It's much easier to offer treatment to somebody than to talk about how they're going to die," he says. "The problem is that, all too often, when a doctor says *treatment*, the patient hears *cure*. But one of my colleagues taught me that when you go through treatment options with a patient, you should always include the option of no treatment—you include it when it might be the best option, so that at least it's on the table."

One disturbing study revealed that even people who are close to death and suffering through futile medical interventions in an intensive care unit do not receive information about options for slow medicine or palliative care. In 2012, the journal *Intensive Care Medicine* published research on the conversations doctors held with family members of very sick patients. These patients had a variety of illness, including cancer and end-stage heart disease. They had already been in an intensive care unit for an average of 12 days and scores calculated from various findings indicated the patients were very likely to die soon, in the hospital, and would never make it home. The investigators recorded the conversations and tallied how often doctors mentioned slow medicine or comfort care as an alternative to continuing aggressive treatments.

Almost half (44 percent) of these doctor-family conferences included no mention of any course other than forging ahead with highly invasive and technological treatment. Ultimately, 72 percent of these patients did die during hospitalization. Surely many endured needless pain and suffering from tests and treatments that had little, if any, benefit.

The researchers wondered what factors might influence whether doctors mention a slow medicine/comfort care option to their patients. They found neither age, diagnosis, days in the ICU nor the calculated likelihood of imminent death could predict whether doctors informed patients or their families of an option for comfort. Doctors who mentioned a slow medicine path were those who personally believed it was the best option. Those who were personally inclined to continue intensive care did not mention any other option.

No Right or Wrong,
Just What the Patient Prefers

Clearly, if individuals want to choose care that aligns with their own values, beliefs and priorities in life, they need to ask direct questions of their doctors and make sure the doctors explain even those options that they personally might not favor. In these circumstances, there is no "right" or "wrong" course. There is only what the patient prefers, in balancing the quality of life with efforts to extend its duration. As the editors of *Intensive Care Medicine* wrote in an opinion piece accompanying the article, "These findings ... raise questions about the process and quality of shared decision-making in the ICU." This is an understatement.

A few years ago, there was a *Frontline* documentary featuring patients in a bone marrow transplant unit in New York City. Along with revealing the suffering caused to patients with virtually no chance of survival, it also provided a disquieting picture of how those often-futile treatments tend to be presented.

Norman Smellie, one of the patients featured in the documentary, was dying from complications associated with his bone marrow transplant, as 25 to 30 percent of patients may. His life partner, Kyimar, was at his side and her distress was evident. She heard Norman say he was tired and wanted to die as peacefully as

Vital Questions to Ask Before Consenting to a Test

- What will the results of the test tell me/the doctor?
- Will that information change the diagnosis, prognosis or treatment options? How?
- What are the burdens of the test in terms of pain, duration and recovery time?
- What can go wrong? What is the possible complication and/or what are the side effects?
- What is the course of action without the test?

possible, if death was his fate. She approached his physician with Norman's request to refrain from further aggressive treatment. In the documentary, you watch the doctor go to Norman's bedside, along with one of his nurses, to discuss this option with him.

The nurse asked, "If something happens and you have trouble breathing, do you want to be put on a respirator to help you breathe?"

Norman nodded.

"You do? Is that a yes?"

"Yeah," Norman confirmed.

The doctor leaned over the bedrails. She told him matter-of-factly that if he was tired and didn't want further treatment, it was all right with her. She concluded, "But you've got to let me know. I don't want to put you through procedures that you don't want to go through, but I don't want to not do the things that are *right* in terms of trying to help you to get better. Okay, Norm?"

Following this interchange, Kyimar, who had been at Norman's bedside almost continuously for two months, reported to the doctor that Norman had clearly expressed to her his desire to sign a Do Not Resuscitate order. The doctor dismissed this information as evidence of ambivalence, and the documentary does not show any attempt to clarify what it was that Norman really wanted.

What happened here? This doctor appeared to regard the conversation as an informed consent for CPR efforts, intubation and artificial ventilation. But was Norman's consent truly informed and independent? Did he fully understand all his treatment options, such as comfort care instead of medical intervention? It does not appear he did. What *did* happen is that a frightened, dying person nodded "yes" to indicate he would like help if he felt he could not breathe. To any person the alternative, fighting for breath, would seem like agony. Plus, the nurse and the doctor told Norman that breathing assistance with a respirator would be the "right" course of action to help him "get better."

Norman received two pieces of misinformation. (1) The only choice for treating his breathing difficulty would be artificial ventilation. And (2) a ventilator could help him "get better." Neither of these is true. If Norman deteriorated to the point of requiring a ventilator, his chance of dying would be increased, irrespective of any mechanical interventions.

Artificial ventilation is hard on dying patients and their families. Patients can no longer speak or take nourishment. If they are alert, a tube down the windpipe is extremely distressful. Patients "buck the machine" and must be sedated to near unconsciousness to tolerate it. Seeing their loved ones in such a condition often contributes to the feelings of stress and grief in the patient's family.

Alternatively, when a dying person becomes breathless, morphine and modest sedation can ease the sense of air hunger and enable a peaceful death without machines, tubes or any sense of suffocation.

Norman continued to deteriorate and was soon moved to the ICU. After two days there, his sister Phyllis confronted the team caring for him, saying, "I have a question. And I would like a straight answer. Is my brother dying? I think I need a straight answer."

His doctor had confided to the interviewer on camera earlier in the segment that she'd never seen anyone survive the kind of complications Norman was facing. But neither she nor anyone else on the team was able to provide a straight answer to his sister when she asked them explicitly if Norman was dying. Instead, they turned the question back to her: "What do you think, Phyllis? What do you think?"

Norman spent four days in the ICU before he died.

It was precisely in response to such muddled and evasive communication that Compassion & Choices drafted and lobbied for the Palliative Care Information Act (PCIA) laws that went into effect in California in 2008 and in New York State in early 2011. The PCIA says that when a disease has advanced to the terminal phase and a patient is unlikely to survive six months, doctors must offer to inform them of this and discuss with the patient treatment options focusing on comfort, in addition to those focused on fighting the disease. Underpinning the law is the belief that patients have a right to know when medical intervention offers only very little chance of prolonging their lives. They need to know that as illnesses advance, aggressive treatments usually offer diminishing returns on the investment of energy, suffering and displacement from the relative comfort of home. And they have a right to learn about palliative therapies that could improve the quality of the time remaining to them.

Today, Norman's doctors would be obligated to provide him with the same information they shared with *Frontline's* viewers: that they had never seen anyone in his condition survive. In New York and California today, doctors treating Norman would be legally bound to reveal to him that palliative treatment could ease his anxiety and relieve his breathlessness and pain. He would not have to fear that refusing treatment would increase his suffer-

Vital Questions to Ask Before Consenting to a Treatment

- What is the goal of this treatment, ie, the expected outcome or response?
- What proportion of people receiving this treatment achieve that goal? In other words, how often does it work for people in my situation?
- If the goal is to prolong life, what is the expected increase in life expectancy? How many months or years?
- What are the risks or side effects? How often do these occur?
- How will this treatment affect my quality of life? What is the frequency, duration and recovery time after each treatment?
- Is there a chance this treatment will make my condition worse?
- What are other treatment options?
- Are there additional options beyond those you have mentioned?
- What will be likely to happen if I decline this treatment, or any treatment?

ing. He would be offered the choice to leave the hospital and die at home with hospice care, or he could choose to be moved to a unit within the hospital devoted to palliative care. The laws Compassion & Choices championed aim for a new standard of care in which doctors present palliative support as an option that is just as "right" for a patient like Norman as are intubation and mechanical ventilation in the ICU.

Despite such laws in both California and New York, I must also confess that there is very little evidence of their desired effect. Physician societies lobbied hard against including in these laws any provisions for accountability or consequences for noncompliance. Thus, the mandate to inform patients of palliative care options in these two states is widely ignored.

We all must instead incorporate the desired effects of the law into our attitude, our questions and our own determination to be fully informed before making any crucial treatment decisions.

Where Did Slow Medicine Come From?

Dr. Turbow, the oncologist and slow medicine practitioner, was right. Some things can't be fixed. Some things shouldn't be fixed. And whether the doctor is willing to face these truths and remain fully present with a patient makes a world of difference in that person's end-of-life experience.

Dr. Turbow's behavior no doubt reflects his mindfulness. I would guess that when he does an intake interview, he looks at his patient instead of pecking away at a computer keyboard. I'd wager he asks open-ended questions rather than jumping ahead to determining which tests to order. He takes the time to listen to patients. Today, the fledgling slow medicine movement aspires to bring that slower-paced, more personal and thoughtful mode of care to everyone.

We've all heard the entreaty: Don't just stand there; do something! But slow medicine often urges the reverse: Don't just do something; stand there. Or better yet, sit there and bear compassionate witness to the patient's experience.

One leading proponent of the slow medicine movement is Dr. Victoria Sweet, associate clinical professor of medicine at the University of California, San Francisco. She is also a prize-winning historian and author of a vivid 2012 medical memoir titled *God's Hotel: A Doctor, a Hospital, and a Pilgrimage to the Heart of Medicine*, and the 2017 follow-up *Slow Medicine: The Way to Healing*.

Dr. Sweet had been a physician for several years when she decided to go back to graduate school for a Ph.D. in medical history. After getting her degree, she could find only one hospital that would hire her part-time: a sprawling complex known as Laguna Honda, in San Francisco, the last almshouse (a charitable residence for the poor, old and distressed) in the U.S. High on a hill overlooking the ocean, with a bell tower and turrets, it looked like a medieval monastery. Occupying 62 acres and hosting 1,178 patients, it had long, open wards harkening back to the time when monks cared for patients. It also had gardens, a greenhouse, an aviary and a barnyard, which aligned with Dr. Sweet's thinking and medical ethos.

Dr. Sweet's initial commitment to Laguna Honda was two months. She stayed for two decades. And during this time, she became a devotee of slow medicine, a phrase she uses to describe her own medical practice, which was uniquely informed by the study she had undertaken for her Ph.D.

The subject of Dr. Sweet's dissertation was Hildegard of Bingen—a 12th-century nun who was an abbess, a visionary and a medical practitioner. Hildegard, too, had written a book, *Hildegard of Bingen's Medicine*, that Sweet describes as thrilling, because it offers an in-depth look at "premodern medicine" that predated, by centuries, the system we have today.

"This book was fascinating because it wasn't the 'eye of newt, toe of frog' medicine we expect from a medieval medical text," Dr. Sweet recalls. "It was real medicine for real patients, but it was based on a completely different model of the body than our mechanical model. Hildegard's idea was that the body was more like a plant than a machine. What's the difference? Someone must fix a machine, but a plant has the power to heal itself. And Hildegard called this power the plant's "greening power" or *viriditas*. Moreover, she believed that the body had its own *viriditas*, and the doctor's responsibility was to nourish it and remove obstructions to it.

As Dr. Sweet says in her 2017 book, slow medicine means "stepping back and seeing my patient in the context of his environment," and providing medical care that is "slow, methodical and step-by-step." One example of this could be taking a conservative approach to treatment, that spares a frail person the pain and risks of more aggressive options and harnesses the body's amazing capacity for healing. Another example may be foregoing an invasive, brutal or disfiguring course of treatment of a terminal illness altogether, in favor of preserving as high a quality of life as possible, for as long as possible.

Doing Slow Medicine, the Second Time Around

The following story comes from someone within our own Compassion & Choices family of professional consultants, social researchers and program developers. Incredibly enough, Rob Gould's personal experience with the death of his mother and father covers the entire spectrum of treatment. First, Rob's family suffers through the dysfunction of intensive treatment, despite its having a very low chance of success. Then, Rob invokes slow medicine to achieve a gentle recovery for his mom. Finally, a slow medicine approach enables his mom to retain bodily integrity, emotional tranquility and personal dignity at the end of life.

Here's Rob's story in his own words:

> My dad had bypass surgery at age 87, but by the time he was 90, he was suffering from heart failure. He'd had several previous emergencies involving fluid in his lungs. He was still living independently with my mother in his hometown on Long Island, New York. At that time, I was living in Miami and my sister was in Washington, DC.

When my mom called to report another emergency, I flew up to find my dad in the ICU. He was not doing well. He was weak and—having suffered from continuous and humiliating bouts of C.dif (inflammation of the colon caused by the bacteria Clostridium difficile) for the past two years—he was now incontinent. During the next six weeks, my sister and I coordinated visits to see him. We conferred with a host of doctors: his internist of many years, a cardiologist and other specialists. Since my dad had survived and returned home after similar scares, we were not surprised when they encouraged us to find a rehabilitation center he could enter upon his recovery and release from the hospital.

There was a brief window of optimism in which Dad started to eat semi-solid food again. But then a day later, he aspirated some of that food, which left him weaker and more compromised than ever. After that, he seemed to improve a bit over the next day or two. The specialists recommended putting a feeding tube in place for him, if he regained enough strength. This seemed the logical choice, if we wanted him to avoid another aspiration as he regained his strength.

It was around this time that Dad's internist told me, "Rob, in all candor, your dad's systems are failing. I'm not optimistic about this." But his was the lone voice of pessimism and, compared with the other doctors, he just seemed like a Gloomy Gus.

When asked about this decision, my dad said, "I'm 91. I want to go home." Right up until the end, he was as mentally sharp as he'd always been, which is to say he was very sharp, indeed. But my mother, aware that she couldn't care for him in this condition, was not encouraging, which depressed him. It was definitely not the most ideal way to cap off a wonderful and loving 58-year marriage. Meanwhile, the specialists, ever confident they could lick every challenge, asked if we had chosen a rehab facility.

During my time in New York, my interactions with Dad were loving but very depressing. He was weak and unhappy and scared. He'd always hated hospitals. Even visiting someone else in the hospital left him with the willies. He was living his nightmare and he was so frustrated that he couldn't "just go home."

More prescient than I about what was coming, Dad asked, "Promise me you'll take care of your Mom." I promised, of course, as I had a hundred times before. I didn't recognize that this time was different.

I went back to Florida but continued to press for constant updates, ready to fly back on a dime if things took a turn in either direction.

A few days later, I got an update. A feeding tube had been inserted. Then another day or so later, there was a new update: Dad would be taken out of the ICU and transferred to a regular hospital room. What good news! Out of the ICU! My sister and I began planning our next respective visits. She'd go up in a few days to be with our parents and I would come the following week to make arrangements for rehab.

Two days later, we each received a call and were told that Dad had died. Mom, thank God, had been with him.

In the immediate wake of his death, we focused on doing everything we could to celebrate his life with the family and friends who had loved him. Then it became necessary to focus on our mom. There was no way she could fend for herself at this point, and we turned to the task of dealing with that. We found an excellent assisted living facility near my sister in Maryland and got her moved in and settled.

It was really only after Mom was moved—almost four months after my father died—that I really began to revisit his decline and death. Why had we never been told how dire my dad's condition really was? Why had we never been told that palliative and hospice care were choices we could make? Why hadn't we learned that in-home support for my Mom was available, so that his homecoming would have been a realistic option? Why had we never been told his statistical chances of surviving with a feeding tube? Why had the specialists and my dad's internist not had a meeting to reconcile their divergent views of my Dad's condition and prognosis? Why hadn't I considered the lone dissenting voice of my Dad's internist?

I had other and tougher questions as well. Why hadn't I figured out that I should never have gone back to Florida? Why had I missed the chance to be with my dad on his last day? He and I had been very close, talking to each other once a week or more for years, with lots of visits as well. I knew he hated what was happening to him. Not just the idea that he was dying, but the pain, helplessness, indignity and impersonality even more. I'd hated it too. Why had I let him down?

So, now I had all these questions, and I was asking them too late to do him—or me—any good. But there was still my promise to Dad that I'd "take care of Mom," right to the end.

Flash forward about six years to when I got a call from Compassion & Choices. I'm a communications and social marketing strategist and they wanted to hire me to help design a consumer campaign around the very question that still haunted me: How can we help people get the care they want at the end of life? The answers to this question were difficult to find, but we got to them in time for me to fulfill my father's dying wish—to take care of my mother until the end.

It was around this time that my mother developed sores on her legs that weren't healing. Her nursing home said she needed to be assessed by a vascular surgeon. I went with her to the appointment because she relied on me to talk to the doctors. The surgeon was a nice guy, very friendly. He examined her, looked at the sores on her legs and told us he could do a simple surgical procedure to improve the blood flow.

The stakes weren't as high as they would be in the future. Now mindful of the pitfalls of an unquestioning attitude, I asked, "Okay, well, are there other options? My mom really doesn't like surgery and that seems like a lot for her to go through at this point." She was nodding in agreement. He conceded that there were some other options but added darkly that they came with a risk.

So, I asked, "What is that risk?"

He said the risk was that she'd lose the leg.

So, I asked him to tell me about some of the other, more conservative options. He mentioned a couple of other choices and I kept on pressing, asking, "Well, are there more conservative treatments?" I really pushed for information on all the different ways we could approach this.

Finally, he came to the fourth or fifth option, telling me, "One thing we could try is something like a sock—you put this gauze wrap around her leg and sometimes that's enough to stimulate the blood flow and it might heal that way. But you'd have to bring her back every week, so we can monitor this and see if it's working or not."

I said, "That sounds like a plan!"

We started that course of action and I learned to put the gauze wrap on my mom and change it. I took photos on my smartphone of the wrapping, and took pictures of the sores, and over the next three weeks we could see that we were making great progress. Finally, on the last visit, the sores were pretty close to being fully healed.

So, that was great. And on that last visit, the doctor looked at her leg and said, "Well, it looks like you won't be helping to send my son to Harvard."

By that time, I'd been working with Compassion & Choices for two years and I was no longer the passive, unquestioning family member I'd been when my dad was dying. My father's death had left me with a lot of scars and a lot of regret over failing to understand what was really going on with him at the end of his life. I was fully aware that most people don't press their doctors for all the treatment options, because people don't know what they don't know. It's not just a fear of questioning the doctor's authority that keeps most people from asking questions—it's not even understanding that there might be other options in the first place. If these alternatives are not presented at the outset, most people have no idea that other, more conservative options even exist.

Ultimately, when my mother was faced with something much more dire than leg sores—when she was diagnosed with cancer of the tongue—my advocacy muscles were strengthened, and I felt fully armed going into conversations with her doctor. We learned she had a tumor, and it was a bad one, that she wouldn't get better without major surgery and that there were no real options besides surgery. So, I understood that the consequences of not doing surgery went beyond the risk of persistent sores or the loss of a leg. Not doing surgery meant, with certainty, that my mom was not going to be surviving for a whole lot longer.

But, I was still able to ask enough questions and provide enough guidance to get a realistic picture of the risks of surgery and the downsides of aggressive treatment, which were disfigurement and the inability to eat. It was very clear to me that the quality of my mother's life—even if it were extended by a few months by having surgery—was going to be horrible. It would be horrible physically and even more so psychologically, because of her particular personality.

My mother's beauty was one of her defining characteristics. A lot of her pride and identity was wrapped up in her physical appearance. Other people might not like the idea of being disfigured, but I instantly understood that it would be beyond devastating for my mother. And she loved to eat. That was a great pleasure for her, and often eating is among the last great joys that remain for someone who is debilitated in nearly every way. This surgery would take that from her.

So, my siblings and I were straight with her. We told her that choosing not to treat the tumor was a valid option, that without surgery her remaining time would likely be shorter, but it would also almost certainly be gentler. She was glad to know she didn't have to submit to painful and disfiguring surgery.

So, she went into hospice. We had a terrific hospice team—an integrated team with social workers, skilled nurses and doctors working with the staff at her nursing home. For the last few months of my mother's life, she really did have great care, with support from my sister and me. We worked together, and my mom did not suffer, and she did not die of suffocation or any other horrible cause of death. And, she died before her cancer could manifest itself in any number of horrifying ways. I grieve for her and miss her, but I'm not suffering from the same anguish I felt after my father died. This time, I don't feel regret or guilt about any aspect of my mother's death.

Rob's experience confirms tenets Dr. Sweet considers essential to the practice of good medicine. Several of these can be summarized in the words of Dr. Francis Peabody, in some lines from his speech to the graduating class of Harvard Medical School, in 1927: *The secret in the care of the patient is in caring for the patient. Medicine is personal: face to face. And when it's personal, it works.* And a final line: *A secret of healing is inefficiency.*

Patience and a Sense of Shared Humanity

It goes without saying that we need more physicians who practice as do Drs. Turbow and Sweet. I'm encouraged by the presence of another compelling advocate of slow medicine, Dr. Dennis McCullough, the author of the 2008 book *My Mother, Your Mother: Embracing "Slow Medicine," the Compassionate Approach to Caring for Your Aging Loved Ones.*

Dr. McCullough has been a family physician and geriatrician for more than three decades. Raised by his mother and grandfather in an impoverished mining community in Michigan, he grew up with a deep allegiance to the underserved.

As a medical student at Harvard, he resisted the path taken by most of his classmates—entering a specialty where performing procedures brings a steady and high stream of income. During his years as a family physician, he helped bring natural childbirth to his rural community in New England. He made house calls whenever elderly patients were unable to visit his office. He acted as a liaison between his local hospital and the major academic center nearby, and he brought medical students to third-world clinics where they served as volunteers. Eventually, an abiding preoccupation with the special needs and complexities of his elder patients led him to become a geriatrician.

A second, deeply personal experience informed Dr. McCullough's advocacy—attending to his own mother during her gradual decline and death. In this book, *My Mother, Your Mother*, he charts this stint of several years. In its opening pages, his mother, Bertha, is 85 and still living independently. In its final chapters, she dies a peaceful death at the age of 92. In the pages in between, McCullough discusses in depth the circumstances that made possible his mother's peaceful death.

Dr. McCullough defines the practice of slow medicine as "using the allotted time health professionals (and families) spend with our aging patients differently and making better, more appropriate decisions more slowly and over a more extended period of time."

He adds, "Slow medicine is not really new in the annals of medicine, but it needs to be retrieved and given prominence again. Many doctors in the trenches are in mourning for the age-old practice of paying deep attention and truly 'attending' that is being squeezed from our complex, fragmented, and technological medical system." He recounts that slow medicine for elders enacts the ancient Tibetan wisdom of "making haste slowly." Such a practice is as much spiritual as medical. It calls for patience and a sense of shared humanity. It will engage patients in tasks inherent in being an elder: "forgiving one another for what cannot be changed, bending flexibly at times of need and holding firmly to shared values and loyalties at other times."

In his book, Dr. McCullough identifies five principles at the core of slow medicine and that inform the end of life. These are:

1. The endeavor to deeply understand the patient, in all his or her complexity, and to acknowledge both the particular losses and specific strengths that emerge during the course of aging

2. An acceptance of the need for interdependence, and the promotion of mutual trust

3. A diligent effort to communicate well and practice patience

4. A commitment to steadfast advocacy

5. A resolve to maintain an attitude of kindness in any situation

One crucial truth is that we cannot realize the benefits of slow medicine if we indulge in denial. As aging or illness advance, we must be willing to accept that, though everything might be fine now, eventually it won't be. We would do well to embrace the wisdom and poignancy in Jane Kenyon's poem, "Otherwise." Kenyon recounts a day of simple pleasures we often take for granted, like rising on "two strong legs," and notes that "it might have been otherwise." Indeed, someday it will be otherwise and holding that truth close to our hearts does two things for us. It causes us to treasure the simple capabilities we exercise every day, and it compels us to make decisions about medical tests and treatments with the understanding that we cannot stave off decline and death forever. And a time will come when the cost of trying to do that is too great to bear.

The more groundwork we do in advance—the candid, hard conversations, the formation of a support team (which McCullough poetically calls a "Circle of Concern"), an honest assessment of a person's vulnerabilities and needs, a realistic anticipation of what might lie ahead—the more peaceful and manageable each stage of decline will be. McCullough does not minimize the effort and deliberation all this entails, but emphasizes that the result is well worth it.

A Laboratory for the Slow Medicine Movement

Dr. McCullough's *magnum opus* in the realm of slow medicine is the retirement community known as Kendal at Hanover, an affiliate of Dartmouth Medical School in New Hampshire. Founded and directed by Dr. McCullough, Kendal has been called a laboratory for the slow medicine movement. Its residents—whose average age is 84—can and often do decline a range of medical interventions, from hospitalization to nutrition and hydration.

The benefits of slow medicine are clear in the gentle course taken by one of Kendal's elderly couples, the Giegs. Charley Gieg already had heart disease, a digestive disorder and the onset of Alzheimer's when his doctors speculated that he also had throat cancer. His proposed treatment plan included biopsies, surgery and chemotherapy. His wife doubted he would be able to weather the course and she feared that aggressive interventions would only hasten his decline.

Journalist Jane Gross wrote about the couple for *The New York Times* in 2008 and noted that, "Such fears are rarely shared among old people, health care professionals or family members, because etiquette discourages it. But at Kendal—which offers a continuum of care, from independent living apartments to a nursing home—death and dying is central to the conversation from Day 1."

Joanne Sandberg-Cook, one of Kendal's nurse practitioners, stayed in touch with Charley's wife, Edie Gieg, throughout his medical consultation in another town. In an email to Mrs. Gieg, she wrote, "I think it is imperative that none of this be rushed!" She urged the couple to resist their doctor's "do-it-now" style and insist on the time to consider the situation realistically and fully.

Ms. Sandberg-Cook asked whether the Giegs would sign on for surgery if Charley were indeed found to have throat cancer. If they wouldn't, then what was the point of a biopsy, which could further weaken his voice, or of enduring anesthesia, which could exacerbate his cognitive decline? Edie Gieg conceded that she shared these reservations and ultimately the couple opted for no further diagnostic tests or invasive treatments. The couple returned to Kendal, where Charley could spend the time remaining to him in relative peace and comfort.

Kendal's intake interview includes questions about whether new residents would wish to receive resuscitation procedures or enter the hospital, and under which circumstances. Brenda Jordan, Kendal's second nurse practitioner, says residents are initially perplexed by the question—"They give me an amazingly puzzled look, like: 'Why wouldn't I?'"

Jordan responds with the statistics reported in the journal *Heart* in 2002. She tells them that, of the few patients in their eighties and nineties who are revived after suffering a cardiac arrest at home, fewer than 2 percent live for one month. Perhaps as a result of knowing these numbers, the vast majority of Kendal residents ultimately indicate a wish *not* to receive CPR.

Gross' *Times* article about Kendal at Hanover concludes with the uplifting testimony of Suzanne Brian, whose father, an 88-year-old resident, chose to discontinue his medication so as not to prolong his decline from congestive heart failure.

"It was my father's choice," Ms. Brian said. "He could have changed his mind at any time. They slowly weaned him from the meds and he was comfortable the whole time. All he wanted was honor and dignity, and that's what he got."

Not all of us may have access to a place like Laguna Honda or Kendal at Hanover. But all of us have the right to control the pace and intensity of our own medical treatment; all of us are entitled to make decisions about our own health care as illness advances and we become frailer and weaker. It is within our power to make an honest assessment of our own life force, our own *viriditas*, and to determine what nourishes and sustains it as well as what diminishes and drains it.

When faced with a new health disorder or exacerbation of an old one, we can assess whether undergoing treatment for it would be worthwhile. Often this decision will be made by weighing the benefits and burdens of each test and treatment: *What will be learned or gained? What percentage of patients respond and achieve some gain in either the quantity or quality of life? What are the burdens of such treatment? Is it painful? Will it sap our energy or have other undesirable side effects? Does it require a lot of time in the clinic or hospital, away from activities that give life meaning and joy? Is the treatment likely to make me sicker, weaker or even shorten my life?*

If the burdens are great and the likelihood of benefit is low, we can refuse to undergo an invasive test or aggressive treatment regimen. We can seek out doctors with a holistic approach to health; who take time to listen, consider and reflect; doctors who are willing to partner with us rather than dictate to us. We can make sure we've done the groundwork and had the important conversations with everyone who matters. This way, when crisis strikes, attitudes don't arise only from the heat of the moment and decisions do not come with pressure and duress.

"'Fast Medicine' is running its lockstep, breakneck course," Dr. McCullough says, "and no one in or out of the system seems to know how to put on the brakes."

It's up to us, the patients and families, to resist the momentum of this runaway train. Only we can make it stop or slow it down. Only we can decide to reach our destination in a different way.

8

Escaping Dementia

My mother-in-law, Virginia, had some diverse character traits. She was both practical and mystical, exotic and provincial. She bore and raised four children, married three times and reunited with her first husband several years before cancer struck him and he needed her care. Her formal training was in nursing but she had investigated the mysteries of psychic healing in Scotland's Findhorn community. Much about Virginia was a paradox, and even some of her own family members never completely unraveled the complexities of her character.

Virginia was open-minded and flexible in just about everything, but she had very specific ideas about growing frail in her old age and losing mental acuity. She didn't want to do it. Virginia lived close by and, perhaps because of the work I did, she always spoke frankly with me about such things.

One such conversation happened in my kitchen, when Virginia was in her mid-seventies. Spry and sharp, she was still driving her own car and even taking sporadic work as an in-home caregiver to augment her retirement income. She was content and stable living alone and caring for herself and others.

But life threw her a curve when she received notice that the apartment building where she had lived for decades was being converted to condominiums. She would have to move. Suddenly a host of difficult questions were on the table. *What would be the best location? How close should she live to each of her four adult children, especially the closest daughter? How long would it be before she was likely to need daily assistance? Was it time to consider a continuing-care community?*

Virginia was unwilling to consider anything other than another single-occupant apartment, as near as possible to the suburban location of the one she had to leave. It was during one memorable kitchen conversation that I asked, "Virginia, what would you think about moving to a location where you could walk to cultural events downtown? Or maybe you'd want to be on a public transportation route, to prepare for when you aren't driving anymore."

"Not driving anymore?" she asked, a little startled.

"Well, yes. Either deteriorating vision or some other problem is likely to mean you won't be driving your own car forever."

"Not me," she answered. "If I can't drive I'll be ready to check out."

"Really?" I asked. "If you could no longer drive a car, you would be ready to die? I can't believe you really mean that. Millions of people lead full lives without driving a car."

"Well, not me."

And that was the end of the conversation.

Shortly thereafter, Virginia moved to an apartment complex just off an eight-lane, pedestrian-unfriendly thoroughfare, with no public transportation and no special senior services available. A few years later, true to the insightful and prudent part of her character, she told us she would no longer be driving and gave up her car. What prompted her decision we don't know, because she never talked about it. Perhaps she had a close call in traffic or just got lost on a shopping trip.

In retrospect, the voluntary loss of driving seemed to announce that Virginia had decided to accept whatever nature had in store for her. She was secure in the knowledge that her life had been full and complete. She seemed to have no fear of death—nor even, anymore, of decline. But what would be the cause of decline? Virginia had no chronic illnesses. She had no reason to seek medical attention and so, for the most part, she didn't. Her approach to her remaining years was the very essence of *laissez faire*.

Early one morning in her 83rd year, about a year after she stopped driving, Virginia made her usual sojourn to the bathroom in the dim light. As she stood at the sink to wash her hands, she noticed one side of her face drooped and one hand felt heavy and weak. "Hmmm," she thought, "maybe a stroke." She phoned the doctor's office and reached an advice nurse who told her to hang up and call 911 immediately.

Virginia, a trained nurse herself, spent a few moments considering her options. She had seen enough of hospitals to know the emergency room was often the entrance to a conveyor belt of tests and treatments, with all their attendant hazards and side effects. That door led to the cold and dehumanizing environment she wished to avoid at nearly any cost. Hospitals meant disorientation and loss of comfortable habits and familiar surroundings. Aggressive treatments carried the risk of medical errors, secondary infections and other harmful incidents. She thought about the fact that if this was a stroke, it could progress. She could even die. She thought about all these things and then she went back to bed.

The next morning, Virginia awoke, looked in the mirror and saw her face was symmetrical again. Her hand felt strong again. "Ah, just a little TIA,"—a transient ischemia attack—she said to herself. If she needed confirmation that she had made the right decision, this was surely it. From now on, *nonintervention* would be her watchword and she hoped whatever ailment or calamity came, it would take her down quick and clean.

That was her hope, but not her fate. Virginia's mental functions steadily diminished and, at age 88, she moved to assisted living. By the time she was 93 she had long since lost the ability to read her beloved *Science of Mind* magazines, and remained confined to the "memory unit" where she slept almost continuously. Virginia became a different person, one who was docile and content to hold a book without reading it, to sit in the presence of loved ones without speaking.

Whether or Not to Become a Different Person

Whether to become a different person—this is the decision everyone with Alzheimer's or other advancing dementia must make. Some, like Virginia, seem to decide, consciously and affirmatively, to let the mind go, along with so many other bodily functions. With this decision, she left behind the woman who had wanted to be alive only if she could think clearly and perform complex tasks like driving a car. Others never make this kind of conscious decision but get blindsided by encroaching dementia. They may deny what is happening to them, blame others for their confusion and slide into a state in which they can no longer decide whether they want to continue living as this other person or not.

Virginia was, for the most part, quiet and docile as a demented person. Her family could think of her as content, if not exactly happy. But many people with dementia become angry and hostile. For their families, the experience hovers between tragic and terrifying and they cannot believe the person their loved one has become is "happy."

Many of the calls we receive at Compassion & Choices are about dementia. We have heard harrowing stories about how dementia devastated entire families. In the following two testimonies, I've withheld last names to protect the privacy of the individuals:

> In the movies, people with Alzheimer's are sweet and childlike and bewildered. Well, that wasn't how it was for us. My father turned into a mad dog. He was the most mild-mannered man before the Alzheimer's—everyone loved him. But he changed into a completely different person: raging at everyone, spitting, cursing. He purposely brought his knee up under my mother's chin while she was crouching by his chair to tie his shoes. It's lucky he didn't break her jaw. This is a man who never lifted a finger against her in forty years. Another time, he threw a bunch of glasses and plates on the floor and then cut the bottoms of both his feet

on the shards. The bloodbath in the kitchen was like something out of a mafia movie.

My mother cared for him at home as long as she could. But she became afraid of him. She was afraid for her own safety in her own home. Everything my parents had went toward keeping my dad in a special, locked-care facility for people with Alzheimer's. — *Sophie K.*

There's no way to describe the hell of advanced dementia. My wife has lost far more than her memories. She's lost everything: all her connections to the people she loves, all her talents, her favorite pastimes and her hobbies, her entire sense of self. It's like a horror story. Do you remember *Invasion of The Body Snatchers*? Her body is still here but it's like a vacant shell.

She's terrified all the time. She doesn't know where she is or even who she is. She doesn't know her own name. Needless to say, she also has no idea who I am. She wakes up in the morning and sometimes she shrieks with fear because it's like a strange man is in bed with her. Can you imagine how this feels to me after all these years?
— *Paul W.*

As these accounts reveal, one of the cruelest aspects of Alzheimer's and other forms of dementia is that they strip individuals of their essential character, along with their memories. Gentle, unassuming people may rage at and physically attack those they love most. Elegant and dignified people may soil themselves without appearing to notice or care. Devoted grandmothers may be indifferent to the most poignant milestones in their own families: births, weddings or graduations. Powerful men who took pride in protecting and providing for their loved ones may be reduced to childlike dependence, clinging to their wives, afraid to be left alone. Or some may become wild and erratic, suddenly seizing a knife or heavy object and striking out.

Many elderly people in America own guns, and these present a heightened risk if the demented person mistakes loved ones or caregivers for strangers or becomes angry or agitated. *The New York Times* columnist Paula Span documented these dangers in her "New Old Age" blog post from May 2018.

Sometimes doctors are forced to employ sedatives and psychotropic medications as so-called "chemical restraints" to prevent those with violent behaviors from harming themselves or others.

Dementia is a huge problem, both for its personal devastation and its impact on society. According to the Alzheimer's Association:

- Alzheimer's has been on a steep rise in the United States. Between 2000 and 2015, deaths attributed to Alzheimer's disease increased by 123 percent.

- One in three seniors dies with Alzheimer's or another form of dementia. Of the estimated 5.7 million Americans with Alzheimer's, more than 96 percent are age 65 and older.

- Alzheimer's disease is the 6th leading cause of death in the United States.

- An estimated 47 million people live with dementia worldwide, and that number is expected to increase to 75 million by 2030, and 141 million by 2050. Dementia due to Alzheimer's disease is estimated to account for 60 to 80 percent of dementia cases.

- Of the top ten causes of death in America, Alzheimer's is the only one that cannot be cured or even slowed.

Happily, the news is not all bad. A recent study of 21,000 people across the United States showed that the dementia rate among people over age 65 fell from 11.6 percent in 2000 to 8.8 percent in 2012. The average age of participants in this study, called the "Health and Retirement Study," was 75. This study focused on people living with dementia, not dying with it. So, it reflects recent progress and is truly good news. The authors attribute the falling incidence to better management of high blood pressure, diabetes and heart disease. Higher education among seniors than was seen even a few years ago also correlates with a lower dementia risk. Although we have no cure nor any effective means of slowing the progression of dementia, we do know that the healthy behaviors that improve overall health and prevent diabetes, strokes and heart attacks also lower the risk of dementia.

Even on the decline, however, Alzheimer's consumes an enormous amount of caregiving resources and often burdens caregivers both financially and emotionally. The Alzheimer's Association reports that:

- In 2018, friends and relatives provided an estimated 18.4 billion hours of uncompensated care to loved ones with dementia, valued at $232 billion.

- Approximately 67 percent of these caregivers are women and about 34 percent are seniors. Of the total, 41 percent have a household income of $50,000 or less.

- An estimated 250,000 children and young adults (in the age range of 8-18) provide care to people with dementia.

- Caregivers are often elderly themselves and their caregiving, in turn, creates its own set of health issues and a secondary set of health-related costs.

- Nearly 60 percent of dementia care providers rate the stress levels associated with caregiving as "high" or "very high." Around 40 percent of these caregivers suffer from depression.

- Due to the physical and emotional burdens of caregiving, Alzheimer's and dementia caregivers had $9.7 billion worth of additional health care costs of their own in 2014.

Dementia and Unwanted/Uninformed
Medical Treatment

Unfortunately, people who face dementia are not immune to a medical system that subjects people to needless tests and treatments. They too are vulnerable to being placed on a conveyor belt of automatic and unwanted medical treatment. As a result, people with dementia often live under treatment for eight to ten years, trapped by a medical system that assumes the primary goal of care is to extend the absolute quantity of life when in fact, few people would choose that course if given the option.

Perhaps the most startling fact is that nine of every ten people living with dementia have at least one invasive medical procedure in the last week of their life. It seems unimaginable. Even those who have been living without recognizing loved ones, without meaningful conversation or lucid thinking for years, will undergo interventions like cardiac pacemaker implantation, hip or knee replacement or other procedures they presumably would refuse if they could assess their situation. Instead of carefully calibrating treatments to the circumstances and previously stated wishes of the person, system-wide habits conspire to prolong the decline to death.

Millions of dementia patients with no hope of recovering mental function receive treatments designed to restore health and vigor. People endure implanted defibrillators, mechanical ventilation, feeding tubes and other burdensome interventions, across years of profound mental deterioration. Usually, these run directly counter to the treatment they would accept if they had the ability to state their preferences. At least, they run directly counter to the vague instruction to "just shoot me," or to similar unrealistic plans people may have proposed when they were of sound mind.

Potentially devastating infections like pneumonia, once called "the old man's friend," or others like urinary tract infection and festering bedsores receive repeated courses of antibiotics to stave off what might have led to a gentle death. This is the fate awaiting countless Americans living with dementia right now, and many more who will develop the condition in the future. I am not suggesting that society should proactively act to shorten the life of people with dementia. This is not about euthanasia. I am merely suggesting that medical standards not assume a goal of life extension for everyone with advanced dementia, so that medicine could yield gracefully to the forces of nature, at appropriate times, and still meet standards of excellence for patient care.

It is important to know that it is possible for mentally competent adults to document their specific wishes for treatment, artificial feeding and other options to be applied on their behalf, should dementia take hold. Whether by video or written statement, documentation today of rational wishes can restore autonomy and dignity to later suffering. This chapter reveals how you might do this.

Early Detection

The essential first step to escape dementia, naturally, is to detect its early signs and understand the future you face. Unfortunately, planning is often complicated and delayed because dementia goes unrecognized and undiagnosed. In fact, only 45 percent of Alzheimer's patients (or their caregivers) report being explicitly informed that they are dealing with dementia.

If there is any chance to escape dementia, you must know for certain it is there, gauge its severity and note the speed of its progression. Success will depend on your ability to recognize the early signs of serious mental decline so that you can take action while still mentally capable. The onset can be subtle and the advance insidious.

Anyone who wishes *not* to become the "different person" of dementia is wise to become alert to the early signs of dementia and track them closely. These may be as benign as an altered sleep pattern and as common as new anxiety, depression or mood swings.

On the other hand, misplacing cell phones or keys happens to almost everyone and can happen more often as we age. While we should not let such lapses frighten us, even a false alarm may serve a purpose if it raises our awareness of genuine warning signs.

Below are some of those genuine warnings. Once these symptoms are present, indulging in denial can make matters worse. The following changes—especially if several occur simultaneously—may indicate the onset of dementia and warrant medical evaluation:

- A memory loss that affects life on a daily basis;
- A new difficulty with problem-solving or planning. It may become more difficult to plan a project, shop efficiently, cook a meal or plan a party;
- Challenges to the performance of routine tasks at home, in the workplace and elsewhere;
- General confusion, especially about what you are doing or why you are doing it. This does *not* include the common experience of being distracted and walking into a room and momentarily forgetting why you came there;
- Compromised ability to decipher visual images and comprehend spatial relationships;
- A persistent struggle to find words when talking or writing;
- Frequent loss of objects, along with an inability to retrace your steps to find them;
- Compromised judgment and an inability to weigh the pros and cons of a decision;
- Inability to concentrate;
- Social isolation. Loss of interest in hobbies, activities and social situations that were previously enjoyable;
- Changes in mood and personality, including apathy and depression.

Any of these symptoms should trigger a thorough medical evaluation. If, in fact, a thorough evaluation or a series of evaluations over time brings confirmation of Alzheimer's or other dementia, people can ask themselves these all-important questions: *"Am I willing to become a different person, perhaps seriously dysfunctional and very different from who I am today? Am I willing to experience substantially diminished mental function, verbal and written communication and conscious spiritual experience?"*

"Yes, I am" is the answer for many, and for them, no escape plan is necessary. They *will* probably want to do everything possible to slow progression of the disease, and that's another reason to diagnose the problem early. A healthful diet, physical and mental exercise, maintenance of social interaction; some believe these, and other habits, may help maintain mental and physical function. The Alzheimer's Association and other organizations have helpful websites and resources for individuals with dementia and their loved ones.

For Those Who Feel Severe Dementia Is Worse Than Death

People who answer, "No, I am not willing to become substantially different as well as mentally, emotionally and spiritually compromised," will need courage and resourcefulness to "outsmart" encroaching dementia and foil its ravages.

Some people regard living with advanced dementia as a fate worse than dying. For them, I'll outline some alternatives which will allow a natural physical decline and death, or will accelerate the timing of death when the threshold of what the individual regards as an acceptable quality of life has been crossed.

The first line of defense is to gather information and begin to think clearly about the future. Whether or not you're confronting early dementia symptoms, there is no downside—and much to be gained—from considering what you would want to happen if serious dementia or other mental incapacity were to set in. After all, dementia has one advantage: it comes on gradually, creating the time and opportunity to act. Sudden catastrophe such as stroke or neurological injury can result in similarly diminished brain function, but with no warning and absolutely no opportunity for prevention of the loss of quality of life.

As with any other disease process, gaining clarity about your own values and priorities is paramount, and is the first step. I recall a married couple with very different perspectives. The husband felt life would be worthwhile only so long as his mental faculties were intact—that is, only if he could think, read, exchange ideas with colleagues and engage in conversation with loved ones. He felt he could sacrifice his physical mobility, but would be ready to surrender his life were his mind to go. His wife had the opposite outlook. She told her husband that as long as she was able-bodied and seemed happy, taking some enjoyment from one moment to the next, he should let her be.

Your line in the sand need not be near that of anyone else. But it's important to consider and discuss precisely where your line is, long before the powers of discernment desert you. Even those who actively decide, or decide by inaction, to "become another person— a person with dementia," may have specific preferences about how far down that road they're willing to go.

Eventually, if no other disease process intervenes to shorten life, progressive dementia renders people unable to walk or feed themselves without assistance. People with advanced dementia no longer recognize anyone, including their family members. Without feeding by spoon or via stomach tube, they quickly become malnourished because they have literally forgotten how to eat and may not feel hunger. They eventually become bedridden, curled in a fetal position, unable to speak or process information. Unless they are fed and treated for infections and other medical conditions, they die of the consequences of inactivity and malnourishment. Therefore, Alzheimer's Dementia is classified as a terminal disease; the downward course is irreversible and ultimately leads to death. When we treat conditions that would otherwise lead to a natural death, we are not so much slowing the progression of a chronic illness as we are prolonging the process of dying from a terminal one.

Other dementias, such as that resulting from the multiple, tiny spots of brain damage (called multi-focal infarcts) caused by cerebral-vascular disease, do not follow the Alzheimer's pattern, but may also lead to profound mental and physical decline. People become incontinent of urine and feces. Immobility leads to muscle wasting and bedsores. Once the breakdown of skin and other tissue begins, it is very hard to reverse the process. Infection turns bedsores into foul, draining wounds. The frequent turning, cleaning and dressing required to tend those wounds can be agonizing for the patient. Patients are often sedated and medicated for agitation or pain, so spend their days in a semi-comatose state.

Outlining the Boundaries of "Acceptable" and "Unacceptable"

Some people with early dementia are so determined not to descend into such a state that they courageously tally all that can be lost, and outline the boundaries of "acceptable" and "unacceptable." If they discuss these with their physician and family and write them down, those left to make medical decisions on their behalf will have these instructions as a guide when that time comes. I don't, for a moment, underestimate the tremendous courage and moral strength it takes for a lively and independent person to consider what a future with dementia might bring. People who fear dementia more than death do, however, find the strength to face the future.

For example, a person may consider whether they would want to receive life-prolonging treatments of any kind in any of the following scenarios:

- I have lost decision-making capacity because I can't think through the benefits and risks of various alternatives. I am often confused or unaware but I can still get out of bed and dress myself, exercise, hold a conversation and do things I enjoy.

- I can no longer concentrate or process information well enough to follow a story, understand a speech or sermon, play a card game, cook a meal, read a book or focus on music that I have previously enjoyed. I get confused or lost if I'm alone.

• I don't get out of bed, bathe or dress myself anymore. I don't have coherent conversations. I can't read, follow a story on TV or recognize and enjoy familiar music. I don't pray, meditate or engage in my former spiritual practice.

• I stare into space and do not respond when spoken to, fail to recognize close friends or relatives, and do not feed myself if food is placed in front of me. I speak rarely and mostly in grunts, moans or single syllables. I am incontinent of stool or urine and do not notice when I am soiled.

• I don't move by myself but lie in a fetal position in bed if not physically lifted into a chair. I don't respond to external stimuli, sounds, sights or touch, except painful ones. I don't recognize any of my family or respond when they speak to me. I don't feed myself but am fed by spoon or stomach tube.

The above scenarios are general guidelines on the course of dementia.

The following detailed list of dementia stages from the California Department of Health Care Services offers more exact information from which one can decide where to draw the line of endurance.

Guide to Determine Alzheimer Disease or Dementia Stages

(based on the CALIFORNIA DEPARTMENT OF HEALTH CARE SERVICES COMMUNITY BASED ADULT SERVICES (CBAS) SCREENING GUIDE)

COGNITIVE IMPAIRMENTS

"Cognitive impairment" is "the loss or deterioration of intellectual capacity characterized by impairments in short- or long-term memory, language, concentration and attention, orientation to people, place, or time, visual-spatial abilities or executive functions, or both, including, but not limited to, judgment, reasoning, or the ability to inhibit behaviors that interfere with social, occupational, or everyday functioning due to conditions, including, but not limited to, mild cognitive impairment, Alzheimer's Disease or other form of dementia, or brain injury."

Stage 1: No cognitive impairment

Unimpaired individuals experience no memory problems, and none are evident to a health care professional during a medical interview.

Stage 2: Very mild decline

Individuals at this stage feel as if they have memory lapses, forgetting familiar words, names or the location of keys, eyeglasses or other everyday objects. But these problems are not evident during a medical examination or apparent to friends, family or co-workers.

Stage 3: Mild cognitive decline

Early-stage Alzheimer's can be diagnosed in some, but not all, individuals with these symptoms. Friends, family or co-workers begin to notice deficiencies. Problems with memory or concentration may be measurable in clinical testing or discernible during a detailed medical interview. Common difficulties include:

- Word- or name-finding problems noticeable to family or close associates
- Decreased ability to remember names when introduced to new people
- Performance issues in social and work settings noticeable to others
- Reading a passage and retaining little material from it
- Losing or misplacing a valuable object
- Decline in ability to plan or organize

Stage 4: Moderate cognitive decline
(Mild or early-stage Alzheimer's disease)

At this stage, a careful medical interview detects clear-cut deficiencies in the following areas:

- Decreased knowledge of recent events

- Impaired ability to perform challenging mental arithmetic, for example, counting backward from 100 by multiples of seven

- Decreased capacity to perform complex tasks such as shopping for groceries, planning dinner for guests or paying bills and managing finances

- Reduced memory of personal history

- The affected individual may seem subdued and withdrawn, especially in socially or mentally challenging situations

Stage 5: Moderately severe cognitive decline
(Moderate or mid-stage Alzheimer's disease)

Major gaps in memory and deficits in cognitive function emerge. Some assistance with day-to-day activities becomes essential. At this stage, individuals may:

- Be unable, during a medical interview, to recall such important details as their current address, their telephone number or the name of the college or high school from which they graduated

- Become confused about where they are or about the date, day of the week or season

- Have trouble with less challenging mental arithmetic, for example, counting backward from 40 by multiples of four or from 20 by multiples of two

- Need help choosing proper clothing for the season or the occasion

- Usually retain substantial knowledge about themselves and know their own name and the names of their spouse or children

• Usually require no assistance with eating or using the toilet

Stage 6: Severe cognitive decline
(Moderately severe or mid-stage Alzheimer's disease)

Memory difficulties continue to worsen, significant personality changes may emerge and affected individuals need extensive help with daily activities. At this stage, individuals may:

• Lose most awareness of recent experiences, events and their surroundings

• Recollect their personal history imperfectly, although they generally recall their own name

• Occasionally forget the name of their spouse or primary caregiver but generally can distinguish familiar and unfamiliar faces

• Need help getting dressed properly; without supervision, may make such errors as putting pajamas over daytime clothes or shoes on wrong feet

• Experience disruption of their normal sleep/waking cycle

• Need help with handling details of toileting (flushing toilet, wiping and disposing of tissue properly)

• Have increasing episodes of urinary or fecal incontinence

• Experience significant personality changes and behavioral symptoms, including suspiciousness and delusions (for example, believing that their caregiver is an impostor); hallucinations (seeing or hearing things that are not there); or compulsive, repetitive behaviors such as hand-wringing or tissue shredding

• Tend to wander and become lost

Stage 7: Very severe cognitive decline
(Severe or late-stage Alzheimer's disease)

This is the final stage of the disease, when individuals lose the ability to respond to their environment, the ability to speak and ultimately, the ability to control movement. At this stage, individuals may:

- Lose their capacity to produce recognizable speech, although words or phrases may occasionally be uttered
- Need help with eating and toileting and be generally incontinent
- First lose the ability to walk without assistance, followed by the ability to sit without support, smile or hold their head upright. Reflexes become abnormal and muscles grow rigid. Swallowing is impaired.

Ron, a friend and associate of mine whose family is currently planning for his future with Alzheimer's, decided to draw his line at Stage 6. He is willing to accept occasional confusion and the inability to do math, so long as he knows who he is and recognizes his family. But he is unwilling to go on if he knows his beloved wife only as a familiar face, has changed in personality or become delusional or suspicious. Ron is perfectly clear on this decision, and he reached this clarity through intimate and courageous conversation with loved ones early in the course of his illness.

Once you achieve this clarity about where to draw the line of endurance, it's crucial to talk about it and document it so that others have no doubt that you've given the matter careful thought. Then, if your own line in the sand comes into view, your family or healthcare proxy can implement the plan.

If you've talked with your family and written your instructions, your family is more likely to feel prepared to follow those instructions than they would if they had no advance notice and no opportunity to discuss your instructions with you. If your family or healthcare proxy differ in philosophy about quality versus quantity of life, they will nevertheless agree on your stated wishes, even if they don't agree with the decision you have made.

From Wishing to Planning

How many times have you heard someone say, "If I'm ever (insert their particular nightmare condition), please shoot me." I've heard this kind of remark more times than I can count when the conversation turns to dementia or Alzheimer's. I've even said something like this myself.

One friend, an avid hiker and outdoorsman, puts an especially fanciful spin on the theme. He likes to say, "I've told my sons and I've even written it in an advance directive: If I'm ever severely demented, take me on a long, last hike. Walk me deep into the woods in the dead of winter. And leave me there."

I understand these spontaneous requests and the sentiment behind them. They are the earnest expressions of people who don't want the last years of their lives to contradict all that went before. They do not want to compromise or violate the person they are or the memories they leave their families. The irony is that, by providing no realistic guidelines around this issue, they are increasing the chance that their worst nightmare will come true. They are placing their loved ones in an impossible situation.

Would a loving mother really ask her family to commit murder? Could any caring son walk an old man miles into the woods—a man who has no memory of requesting anything like this—and leave him, confused and terrified, to die of hypothermia?

"Just shoot me." "Leave me on an ice floe." These are really ways to say: *Find a way to make sure I don't linger for months or years in a demented state, unable to think, talk or feed myself. I'd rather die than let that happen. Please find a way to help me escape.*

It's a common wish. But a wish is not a plan. We owe it to the ones we love not to leave them with only wild, unrealistic instructions. We owe it to them to lay out a realistic plan to honor our wishes and values under dreaded circumstances.

No one will be at liberty to shoot us and no one will abandon us to the elements. And when it comes to mental deterioration, even hard-won laws authorizing medical aid in dying will be of no assistance. Medical aid in dying is for people who are both mentally capable and terminally ill, with no more than six months left to live. Alzheimer's Disease *is* classified as a terminal illness, as people do eventually die as a result of the disease. But when Alzheimer's patients are in their final six months, they are long past being mentally capable. And those in the early phases, with the ability to make medical decisions, are probably not within six months of death.

Some people are unaware and often disappointed to learn that dementia patients don't qualify for medical aid in dying. But the hallmark of medical aid in dying is respect for the agency of the dying person. It does not confer autonomy or decision-making authority upon anyone else. Thus, it is not an option for people with early dementia who are mentally capable but not terminally ill, nor for people in late dementia who are terminally ill but not mentally capable.

Therefore, escaping dementia means being resourceful and creative in our planning and assertive in the information and instructions we impart to those who love us. Preparedness falls into two categories: 1) The plans and healthcare decisions that can be made while a person is still alert and competent to make healthcare decisions for themselves, and 2) The plans for shortening the period of severe mental impairment caused by dementia, stroke or other catastrophe that renders an individual unable to care for themselves or make decisions.

In other words, what can you do to instruct and empower surrogates, to provide them with a plan more realistic than *just shoot me*? These plans and the conversations they require are hard but necessary.

If you wish to navigate your own or a loved one's cognitive decline with common sense, integrity and compassion, there are concrete, legal steps any one of us can take to keep the final phase of life from going past our "line in the sand."

REALISTIC PLAN #1:

Decline or Withdraw Life-Sustaining Medical Treatments

This option is what I have heard one expert in end-of-life care, Dr. Joanne Lynn, call "creative collaboration with the forces of nature." This means taking advantage of natural events and illnesses as they arise. Capable individuals in the early stages of Alzheimer's disease and dementia, as well as their providers and caregivers later, may decline medical intervention and invite a peaceful death by following their or the patient's belief that the alternative to death—"life" (maintained at any cost)—is the equivalent of torture. When we have reached our "line in the sand" and it's time for our lives to come to a natural close, we do not have to accept everything medical technology has to offer. We may decide that aggressive or even standard medical intervention would merely keep us on a path of increasing debility and suffering, and we may instead choose to graciously decline.

If you decide to refuse life-sustaining measures while you are still mentally capable, this can be done any time and for any rational reason, including an imminent descent into dementia. Often people do not realize it is legal to forego or discontinue any medical treatment, including those that would sustain life. If a person with diabetes makes a rational decision to stop insulin and succumb to a diabetic coma, this is permissible. If a person's heart beats only with electronic pacing and he wants to deactivate the pacemaker, this is also permissible. If a person contracts pneumonia and decides not to fight it with antibiotics, no one can force her to take the medication.

Any plan to decline or discontinue medical treatments and invite a peaceful death should include discussion with loved ones, as well as trusted confidants like physicians and clergy. A hospice program or other palliative care provider should be enlisted to manage any distressing symptoms that may arise after a treatment is refused or withdrawn.

An important part of this plan is to prepare for the possibility that cognitive impairment might come from a stroke or other sudden event, or that dementia might advance swiftly enough to preclude self-determination. Similarly, preparation is also necessary for those who decide to allow dementia to progress beyond the point of their competence to refuse treatment. These people will want to instruct others to withhold treatment when their "line in the sand," that they have previously decided on and discussed, is reached.

Make Sure Your Advance Directive Is Strong

To prepare for any of the above possibilities, you will need to put a plan in place for others to oversee once you've lost mental capability. You specify instructions in documents with the official titles of Advance Directive, Living Will, and Durable Power of Attorney for Health Care (also called a Health Care Proxy in some states).

As I outlined in the "Limits of an Advance Directive" box at the end of Chapter 2, these documents are not as powerful as many people believe them to be and doctors routinely ignore or override them. But they do serve an important function as evidence of your desires and intentions. Family members are more likely to succeed in honoring your wishes when armed with an advance directive that documents your desires and corroborates their instructions to physicians.

One very effective way to memorialize your preferences and instructions is with a video recording. This is easy, now that cell phones have video recording capability, and, in my experience, it is harder to override instructions presented in this way than it is to ignore a piece of paper. (See "Creating a Video Supplement to Your Advance Directive" at the end of this chapter.)

In Oregon, I had the privilege of assisting State Senator Robert Shoemaker as he fought to include a dementia provision within the standard advance directive form. Most advance directives become effective only when a mentally incapable person becomes permanently unconscious or terminally ill, which severely limits applicability of the document. Senator Shoemaker wanted the standard advance directive to apply in situations of advanced dementia as well.

In 1993, the advance directive was still controversial, and the senator's proposal to include dementia as a condition to trigger instructions about life-sustaining treatments was ground-breaking.

I recall one of his senatorial colleagues coming to my Senate office to condemn the Health Care Decisions Act as an affront to God. When he called the bill "heresy," I reminded him that the United States is not a theocracy. People should be allowed to follow their own moral compass, and it isn't the place of our government to enforce any religious doctrine. He left my office in a huff and registered a complaint against me for insubordination, even though he wasn't my supervisor. This was the first time I formally defended individual liberty against those who would use the government to impose their religious beliefs on others.

Since then, other states have also put this dementia provision in place. But even in states where dementia isn't officially recognized in advance directives, adding such a provision as an addendum to your advance directive can be invaluable as a guide for families, healthcare professionals, caregivers and proxies. Below is a version of the suggested Dementia Provision on the Compassion & Choices website. There you will find the most updated version for download.

Addendum: Dementia Provision

I, _____,

am creating this document because I want my health care representatives/agents/proxies, medical providers, family members, caregivers, long-term care providers, and other loved ones to know and honor my wishes regarding the type of care I want to receive if I develop an advanced stage of Alzheimer's Disease or other incurable progressive dementia.

Under the conditions of advanced dementia, including my inability to communicate rationally with loved ones or caregivers, and/or my physical dependence on others for all aspects of bodily care, continuing life would have no value for me. In those conditions, and if my condition is unlikely to improve, I would want to die peacefully and as quickly as legally possible to avoid a drawn-out, prolonged dying that would cause unnecessary suffering.

For this reason, if I have advanced dementia, and I am unable to feed myself due to advanced dementia, I want the following to apply (initial each option that represents your wishes):

_____ To receive comfort care only, focused on relieving any suffering such as pain, shortness of breath, anxiety, or agitation. I would not want any care or treatments that would be likely to extend my life or prolong the dying process. This includes life-sustaining measures like cardiac pacing, cardiopulmonary resuscitation and mechanical ventilation.

_____ In the event of an acute infection, I do not wish to be treated with antibiotics and/or antimicrobials in any form but with aggressive pain and symptom relief only, while the illness takes its natural course.

_____ If I lose the ability to speak for myself and my Advance Directive is being taken into consideration as written, I also would like it to be clear that if I am currently receiving any medications or treatments that are likely to extend my life or prolong my dying process, I would like those stopped.

_____ I request that food and fluids in any form, including spoon-feeding, be stopped if, because of dementia, any of the following conditions occur:

- I appear indifferent to food and being fed.
- I no longer appear to desire to eat or drink.
- I do not voluntarily open my mouth to accept food without prompting.
- I turn my head away or try to avoid being fed or given fluids and am clearly repelled by food or fluids.
- I spit out food or fluids.
- I cough, gag, choke on or aspirate (inhale) food or fluids.
- The negative consequences or symptoms of continued feeding and drinking, as determined by a qualified medical provider, outweigh the benefits.

_____ If the above statement regarding food and fluids goes into effect for any of the above listed reasons, and as a result I begin to experience delirium, agitation or hallucinations, then I would like my medical team to provide palliative sedation in order to avoid suffering until death occurs.

· · ·

I want the instructions in this provision followed even if the person who has the right to make decisions for me and/or my caregivers judge that my quality of life, in their opinion, is satisfactory and I appear to them to be comfortable. No matter what my condition appears to be, I do not want to be cajoled, harassed, or forced to eat or drink. I do not want the reflexive opening of my mouth to be interpreted as giving my consent to being fed or given fluids or misinterpreted as a desire for food or fluids. I have given considerable thought to this decision and want my wishes followed.

Before I am admitted to a long-term care facility, I want that facility to affirm its willingness to honor

these instructions. If the long-term care facility where
I already reside will not honor these instructions, I
want to be transferred to one that will.

Note this is a standard form and does not include your particular "line in the sand" criteria. The form's language describes very severe cognitive decline and you may not wish to go that far down the dementia path. I recommend crossing out any language you don't want and replacing it with words that describe your own "line in the sand."

Your Wishes and Who Will Carry Them Out

Another document, "My Particular Wishes," can also be found on C&C's website. It lists specific interventions that you may decide, in advance, to decline or discontinue if you are in a state of dementia and would not want your life prolonged. These include dialysis, drugs to stimulate the heart and circulation, antibiotics, replacement fluids, nutrition and hydration and other organ system support. Declining any treatment will, of course, produce the symptoms of the untreated disease, which is why it is so important to request the care of hospice or a palliative care program. Stopping kidney dialysis will produce itching and weakness as levels of uric acid and other byproducts of metabolism rise; stopping cardiac drugs may lead to shortness of breath; declining antibiotics for pneumonia will allow fever and lung congestion to progress. These symptoms are all treatable, but a healthcare team should be in place and prepared to provide timely and effective comfort care.

Planning to withdraw or withhold medical treatments means someone else, a trusted surrogate decision-maker, will probably have to put your plan into effect. When the time comes to decline antibiotics for a urinary tract infection, for example, you may be incapable of making the decision yourself. Even if you are still playing a decisive role, doctors and others will want to know your decisions are confirmed and supported by your family, or by the person designated to speak on your behalf once you no longer can.

So, it is not enough to be clear about your wish to decline medical therapies at some specified point. It's essential to assess whether family members, friends and especially the person you name as the surrogate in your advance directive can honor them. When dementia patients are past the point of advocating for themselves, it will fall to others to decline or discontinue life-prolonging measures—including antibiotics, feeding tubes or even spoon-feeding for nourishment and hydration—when the opportunity arises for "creative collaboration with the forces of nature." One of the most crucial actions you can take is to name the person who will serve as a surrogate decision-maker on your behalf. Many people feel compelled to designate a family member as their proxy but this is not necessarily the best choice. A friend, neighbor, colleague or advisor may be a better choice for some.

A colleague of mine has an anecdote that illustrates this point. "If the day ever comes when my mind is gone, and another person has to make medical decisions for me," she said, "I don't want anyone consenting to antibiotics or heart treatments. I would want medical treatment withheld. But when I told my husband this, he said, 'I'm sorry, honey. But I just wouldn't be capable of that.'"

"My sister, on the other hand, would have no problem with it," she added, laughing. "So, I've designated my sister as my legal healthcare proxy instead of my husband." And that's why it's important that we have these conversations while we can. If we want to ensure that our choices are respected, we have to know where our loved ones stand.

REALISTIC PLAN #2:
Decline food and water

When there is no life-sustaining treatment like a heart pacemaker, insulin or antibiotics to decline or discontinue, people on the verge of catastrophic decline may choose instead to stop eating and drinking to hasten their death. In the medical community, this is called "VSED"—Voluntary Stopping of Eating and

Drinking. This is a legal option, and if a mentally capable person decides to refuse nutrition and hydration, no one can force them to do otherwise. Force feeding, or insertion of a feeding tube without consent, amounts to assault, battery and the violation of bodily integrity of another person. You have probably heard of prisoners going on hunger strikes and being forcibly fed. Those circumstances are very different because the civil liberties of prisoners have already been suspended.

The fact that VSED is legal doesn't mean no one will try to interfere with your decision to follow this plan. You will need to create a support network of people who will honor your decision. In addition to writing down or recording your intentions, it's a good idea to talk with loved ones early and often about what you expect from them, to enable your plan to come off without a hitch. A VSED plan also calls for conversation with family and physicians, genuine efforts to enlist their support and prior arrangements being made for good palliative care during the process.

Many people are surprised to learn that abstaining from food and drink is anyone's prerogative, that it does not usually cause great discomfort and that palliative medical care is available to manage symptoms, like dry mouth or agitation. Death does not come by starvation, but by dehydration. Kidneys fail and toxins build up, including some that actually have an anesthetic effect. Hunger does not last long and thirst is easily managed with glycerin swabs to the mouth and lips. Hospice care usually includes mild sedation or morphine after the first few days of VSED.

Depending on the fluid load in a person's body at the beginning of VSED, the process may take as long as 14 to 20 days. The average duration is much shorter—5 to 8 days. Of course, all preparations, family conversations, advance directives, instructions regarding medical care and palliative or hospice services must be in place before a person begins VSED.

Ethyl, at age 99, was a woman with no interest in seeing her 100th birthday. Her multitude of chronic ailments had recently escalated, and each one contributed to the misery of the others.

Together they compromised her mobility and her ability to read, play cards and enjoy the company of friends.

The final blow came when Ethyl realized her mental acuity was starting to decline. She found tasks like balancing her checkbook beyond her ability, and it frightened her badly when she went for a short walk one day and could not find her way home. She desperately wanted to avoid further mental decline or full dementia. Ending her long and fruitful life while she could still make decisions for herself seemed like the reasonable and practical option.

Although Ethyl lived in Oregon, she did not have a prognosis of six months or less to live, so she was not eligible for medical aid in dying. So, she decided to stop eating and drinking. She had little appetite anyway and felt this would be a natural and peaceful way to die. She sought and obtained the support of her family, her friends and her assisted living facility.

Hospices typically regard a person who has stopped eating and drinking as having a terminal condition; once a person has begun to implement this decision, they are expected to die within six months, thus making them eligible to receive hospice services. Ethyl enrolled in a hospice program that would care for her in the home she had known for years. When all was in place, Ethyl enjoyed a carefully chosen last meal and then began VSED. She stayed alert for days and entertained the staff with stories from her long, vibrant life. Ethyl was much loved, and the staff doted on her during this time.

On the sixth day, she surprised everyone by asking for coffee. Delighted that she had apparently reconsidered and abandoned her plan, the staff brought her a tray with cookies and other goodies, in addition to the coffee, and excitedly placed it before her.

"No," she said, disappointing them. "I don't want all that. Do you have a Q-tip?"

Then she slowly dipped the cotton swab in the coffee and rubbed it on her lips. "Ahh, that tastes good," she declared. "But that's enough. I just wanted to taste coffee one more time." Ethyl slipped into a coma that night and died a day later.

Sometimes, as a person begins to lose consciousness, they may forget their decision to abstain from food and water. If a person is only intermittently aware of having chosen VSED, then honoring their intention to not eat or drink may not be possible. Sometimes, being reminded is enough to enable a person who is temporarily confused to stay with their intention. One woman who was a client of Compassion & Choices' consultation service declined food and water without difficulty for three days, but on the fourth morning she asked for a big breakfast. The caregiver wasn't sure what to do, so she called for advice. A member of the consultation team went to visit with the client and ask about her well-being. The client said she felt wonderful and wanted a big breakfast.

The consultant asked, "Well, do you remember three days ago, you told us you wanted to stop eating and drinking because of your illness?"

And she said, "Oh, yes! I forgot all about that! Never mind then, I don't want that breakfast!" And she laughed. This woman quickly reaffirmed her decision when gently reminded of it.

REALISTIC PLAN #3:
Accumulating Life-Ending Medication

I offer the story below with the caveat that it is "realistic" to only the most resourceful and determined among us, and that it requires great care not to put anyone "assisting" us in jeopardy. I would also draw a clear distinction between what a person may want to consider for themselves personally, and what should constitute public policy. Causing one's own death, or attempting to do so, is not a crime in any state. That is as it should be. I believe the best public policy is to create a regulated safe harbor from the "assisting" prohibition, when a person is both mentally competent and terminally ill. I would not advocate an expansion of the eligibility criteria for state-authorized medical aid in dying as a matter of public policy.

Sandy Bem, a brilliant feminist scholar, developed Alzheimer's at age 65. Sandy was a professor emeritus of psychology at Cornell University in Ithaca, New York. She was the director of Cornell's Women's Studies Program and a pioneer in gender studies, known for her intellectual prowess and her capacity for original thought. It was especially devastating for her to experience the cognitive impairments of dementia. The account of her decline and her response to it was featured in *The New York Times Magazine* in May of 2015.

Sandy told her neurologist early on that she did not intend to let Alzheimer's consume her. "I want to live only for as long as I continue to be myself," she said during her first consultation with him. In response, her physician shared some personal information with her, the fact that his own mother had suffered from Alzheimer's. Hoping to change her plan, he suggested that by documenting her own experience of the disorder, Sandy could offer another valuable contribution to the world.

Sandy appreciated his suggestion but would not be deterred. She was forthright and unequivocal about her plan to end her life while she was still able to make a considered decision and act on it. She shared her resolution with her inner circle of family members and close friends. None of them tried to dissuade her; they asked only that she choose a gentle method. Sandy readily agreed to this. "What I want," she wrote in her journal, "is to die on my own timetable and in my own nonviolent way."

Sandy had been separated from her husband Daryl for 15 years, though they remained friends. Now they grew close again. He became her companion and accompanied her to medical appointments.

While planning her demise, Sandy consulted a book describing short-acting barbiturates like Nembutal and Seconal, the same class of drugs commonly used by veterinarians to put animals down. The *Times* reported: "Sandy thought pentobarbital [the drug's generic name] was what she was looking for. It was reliable, fast-acting and—most important to her—a gentle way to die." Pentobarbital in large doses causes swift but not sudden unconsciousness and then a gradual slowing of respiration. She ordered the drug from a foreign supplier and within a few weeks it arrived in the mail.

Two events helped Sandy decide exactly the right time to take this medication. The first was when she experienced uncertainty about how she was related to her daughter. The second was when she became unsure of what to do in response to her feeling of hunger. She had the feeling but did not connect it with a desire for food. To her, these developments signaled nature's way of shutting down her life, both mentally and physically. That was when she decided it was time to act on her plan.

During her last day, Sandy unearthed an email she had sent Daryl months earlier, testifying to her intention to die when she chose to and to the fact that no one had influenced or assisted her in this capacity. She went for a walk with Daryl in the beautiful Fall Creek Gorge. She watched her favorite movie with him for the last time. And then, with her inner circle gathered at her home— forming, in the words of her best friend Karen, *a loving net around her*—she said her final goodbyes, drank the Nembutal with some wine and drifted off in her bed with her husband beside her.

Afterward, NPR aired a story about Sandy in which the journalist Alix Spiegel noted, "The relatives and friend I spoke to agree that something in this process made dealing with Sandy's death much easier."

Her daughter, Emily Bem, echoed this assessment. "This is going to sound really funny, but I wouldn't have had it any other way," she told NPR. "It made it less like a grieving process and less like a sort of horrible thing that had happened, and more like something that made sense and felt right and actually had some joy to it in its own way."

The Difficult Question of Timing

No matter what a person's specific plan might be, timing is the crucial question. No one wants to die prematurely, while still able to do things central to life's joy and meaning. Most people consider life good, so long as they can do things like connect with others, share companionship, enjoy stories and music, savor food, explore books and art, pray or engage in other spiritual practices. But people who want to avoid dementia need to act on their plan while still alert, aware and capable of voluntary action. They are rightly afraid that waiting too long could trap them in dementia's prison.

The public first became aware of this difficult and extremely personal question of timing during the era when Dr. Jack Kevorkian was intentionally and recklessly creating controversy. Janet Adkins, the first person to die in the back of Kevorkian's Volkswagen bus, had very early dementia. An avid hiker, adventurer and outdoorswoman, she was still quite functional, both mentally and physically, when she chose to die at age 54. She reportedly played a game of tennis with her son shortly before her chosen time of departure. Her function was still high, but she perceived dementia closing in and she abhorred the idea of losing her mind. Thus, she died relatively early in the course of her illness. I, like many others, hope and believe I would have made different choices for myself in the same scenario.

Her husband, Ron Adkins, sent a heartfelt letter to the Alzheimer's Association, expressing his support for her decision and stressing the importance of open dialogue. Extracts from this letter are included below:

> My wife, Janet Adkins, was excited by life. She was a woman of many ideas and interests. She was a talented musician and an avid reader. She liked pushing the limit and trying new things, such as trekking through Nepal.
>
> When she was diagnosed with Alzheimer's disease at age 53, she was devastated. She weighed the options of letting the disease take her mind and body or exiting early with the assistance of a doctor while her intellect was still intact. We had openly discussed end-of-life issues, and her choice was not to let the disease progress...

We made an informed decision and a personal choice, one that was right for Janet. Most importantly we openly discussed end-of-life issues together as a family. I encourage others to do the same.

Certainly, people should not have to make their decisions in silence and isolation. An open heart and non-judgmental attitude are great gifts we can give to those looking toward a future with dementia and trying to plan for it. People's most dearly held values are as different from each other as one person is from the next. Open, loving dialogue can help people sort through what, exactly, they are unwilling to lose and how to discern when that loss is imminent.

When Gillian Bennett—an 84-year-old psychotherapist in the early stages of dementia—confronted these questions, she did so with her husband of 57 years by her side. From the vista of her home on Bowen Island, off the coast of British Columbia, Bennett reflected on their adventures together, her lifetime of travel, philosophy and psychology and all that would be lost as her mind deteriorated. Gillian—like Sandy Bem—was unwilling to let the disorder take the most cherished characteristics of her personhood. And like Sandy Bem, she obtained her own supply of barbiturates to avoid that fate.

Gillian documented her final thoughts on her website, Deadatnoon.com. There she left a public note explaining her own decision to die at noon on a late summer's day.

> August 18, 2014—I will take my life today around noon. It is time. Dementia is taking its toll and I have nearly lost myself. I have nearly lost me. Jonathan, the straightest and brightest of men, will be at my side as a loving witness.
>
> I have known that I have dementia, a progressive loss of memory and judgment, for three years. It is a stealthy, stubborn and oh-so reliable disease … Dementia gives no quarter and admits no bargaining … Ever so gradu-

ally at first, much faster now, I am turning into a vegetable …

Each of us is born uniquely and dies uniquely. I think of dying as a final adventure with a predictably abrupt end. I know it's time to leave and I do not find it scary.

We do not talk much about how we die. Yet facing death is thoroughly interesting and absorbing and challenging … I think I have hit upon the right choice for me.

I have talked it over with friends and relatives. It is not a forbidden topic. Anything but.

I have had a husband beyond compare, and children and grandchildren who have outstripped me in most meaningful ways. Since I was seven I have had wonderful friends, whom I did and still do adore.

Today, now, I go cheerfully and so thankfully into that good night. Jonathan, the courageous, the faithful, the true and the gentle, surrounds me with company. I need no more.

It is almost noon.

A Steady Decline and Attempts to Intervene

In a way, my mother-in-law, Virginia, ended up timing her own death, too. Her condition steadily declined during her eight years in assisted living. Gradually, she walked about and read less. She lost interest in personal hygiene and didn't bathe or brush her teeth unless her daughter was there to insist she do so. We celebrated birthdays at her favorite restaurant, where she would eat but not speak.

Her needs eventually became great enough that she moved into the facility's memory unit where doors were locked, and she could not wander or get lost. At first, she was eager to walk outside and around the grounds with us but she stopped wanting to go outside a few months before she died. She had always enjoyed mealtime, but she lost interest in food—first with going to the dining area, then with getting out of bed to eat, and finally in eating anything at all. She slept almost continuously, rousing herself for a few moments when we arrived and then drifting back to sleep.

As often happens, Virginia had an episode of energy and lucidity shortly before she died. On that day, she accepted my husband's invitation to walk outside. Once there, she was enchanted by every aspect of nature around her. She exclaimed over the beauty of the fall leaves, the bark of trees and birds at the feeders. She said to her son, "You'll never forget this day, will you?" And he won't.

After that day, she did what used to be called "turning her face to the wall." A vivid description, the term should really come back into use. Virginia stayed in bed and could not be coaxed out. She lost all interest in food or drink. One day, as we sat at her bedside, the aide came in to try and entice her to eat. She had not stirred, and we thought she was asleep. But she answered his cheery attempts to lure her to a meal with two words, spoken louder than any I'd heard from her in years, "Go away." Her four children talked among themselves and agreed not to intervene in the natural process that seemed to be unfolding.

At least, they thought they had agreed. But in a testament to how difficult it is to abstain from medical intervention even when a family talks and agrees on a plan, when Virginia developed a fever, she was taken to urgent care and treated for a urinary tract infection. Several days later, a nurse requested consent to start a trial of appetite stimulants, to see if Virginia could be led to eat. This time, her four adult children decided in concert to decline. Soon her immobility and malnutrition created bed sores, and when these got bad enough to cause discomfort, the family and professional caregivers decided it was time to seek a hospice referral.

Virginia stayed in bed, receiving no medical treatment except for opiates to dull the discomfort of her bedsores. At age 96, a full

15 years after passing the "not driving" milestone that she had originally wanted to herald the end of her life, she slipped away quietly in the middle of the night. Her family is comfortable that she went at the right time.

Fortunately, like Virginia, you can plan for a dignified death with dementia by identifying your line in the sand, documenting your preferences, making sure you have a strong health care proxy who knows your values and ensuring that all those who will be around at the time of your death will support the proxy in honoring your values. I imagine that you have the fortitude this takes because you are taking the time to read this book.

However, unless we bring the question of how one dies with dementia to the forefront of mainstream dialogue and discussion, the majority of people with dementia will continue to live for eight to ten years being subjected to tests and treatments that are inconsistent with their values and priorities. There may be no greater imperative for aging Americans than to protect themselves and their loved ones from the anguish of lost autonomy in the face of this devastating condition. Because so few people articulate the level of treatment and intervention they would want during their experience with dementia, many endure the irreversible loss of every mental and bodily function long after they intended to have their life end altogether.

That's why I am grateful that Compassion & Choices is tackling the challenging and taboo topic of how to support people with dementia in their quest to die a natural death.

C&C's dementia initiative has the potential to ignite a transformative shift in how every American conducts their end-of-life planning, and to foster meaningful dialog that will enable families and loved ones to apply a person's values and priorities at their life's end. This preparation will surely help those closest to us prepare for whatever lies ahead with compassion, candor, fearlessness and true peace of mind.

Creating a Video Supplement to Your Advance Directive

In your advance directive documents, perhaps you have specified a desired course of treatment to be followed by healthcare providers and caregivers, and shared these with your doctors, your family and your healthcare proxy. As discussed throughout this book, these documents are severely limited. Videotaping a personal message about your wishes can greatly enhance their actual impact on your end-of-life experience.

This recording, showing you in sound mind, expressing your well-thought-out priorities and wishes, will have an immediacy and authentic tone far stronger than any signed and witnessed form. It's still a good idea to complete a witnessed advance directive, but a video is likely to be far more informative and useful to your healthcare proxy and your loved ones.

Preparing to make a video

• **Go digital.** For making a video recording, it's easiest to use a computer, tablet or smart phone, all of which have built-in recording capability. You can record yourself, or have someone else hold the cellphone or digital camcorder for you. If you are technologically challenged, ask someone knowledgeable to help you get started. This could be your local cellphone store clerk, an Apple store employee, your neighbor's kid, a how-to video on YouTube or a librarian.

• **Break it up, if necessary.** The video does not have to be long, and it's probably better to stay at 5 minutes or less. This will make a compact, impactful message. But if you sense your video is going to run longer than ten minutes, plan to record it in multiple sections or separate files since long files can become hard to manage.

• **Make a list of what you want to cover.** In this video, stay on the topic of your values, beliefs and priorities regarding the quality of life and experience of dying as much as possible. Making a list of what you want to cover in the video before you start recording can help you be thorough and concise. Keep your notes nearby during your recording to make sure you don't leave out any important points.

• **Do a short practice recording.** Use this practice recording to make sure the video's sound and lighting are adequate.

The content of the video

• **Start the recording with a greeting.** In the greeting, you should state your name and age, and the day and year of the recording. Maybe add a line or two about why you are making this recording, such as, "You have my advance directive, but this video is about what I care about most at the end."

• **Don't stress.** If you stumble over words or fumble with your papers, don't worry—there are no critics judging this performance. Just keep going, speaking from your heart. Remember that you can always press STOP and re-record.

• **Use your values as a starting point.** As you list what matters most to you in life, you can reference your living will document in which you specified the medical interventions and treatments you do and do not want to receive if your physical condition is dire and unlikely to improve. You might describe how you came to these decisions and how they reflect your most cherished values.

• **Emphasize what matters most.** If there is an event or procedure you feel especially strong about, make sure to highlight it. For example, "I want a gentle, calm death. I do not want to have a tube put down my throat to keep me breathing." Or, "I believe putting myself in God's hands means trying every possible procedure to keep me alive. I don't want anyone to give up on me if an emergency lands me in the hospital." You can look into the camera and pause after outlining an especially important direction to emphasize your point.

• **Fill in the gray areas.** An advance directive goes into effect only if you are incapacitated and unable to speak for yourself. The instructions usually apply only to a person imminently dying or permanently unresponsive. But you may wish to clarify, "Don't wait until I am deemed close to death, absolutely brain dead or comatose to carry out my wishes for a peaceful death. If I am severely compromised and unlikely to regain my ability to _____ (talk to you; recognize you;

respond to you, etc.), I consider my life over. Do not wait too long to put my wishes into effect."

• **Make it personal.** If you have specific thoughts about your personal "line in the sand" after reading over the dementia stages in this chapter, articulate them in this video. Try to use specific and personal references such as, "If I no longer recognize my beloved grandchildren with at least a smile, then do not work to prolong my life." These specific examples will help your proxy understand your thoughts.

• **Quality of life guidance.** If there are some "good to know" quality of life contributors that you want your proxy to remember at the end of your life—"I love opera music but hate Carmen," or "Please don't have any fragrant flowers in my room"—remind them of these in this video.

• **End with a thank you**. Thank your proxy and doctors for viewing this video and attending to your wishes.

• **Review your video.** Make sure you watch your video once you've finished recording, to make sure you've covered all the points on your list.

Safekeeping the video

• **Save and name the video(s):** Joe Smith's Advance Directive Video, January 8, 2019, 15 minutes total, Part 1 (if necessary).

• **Copy the video.** A removable thumb or flash USB drive that can be stored in your "important papers" file along with your other end-of-life documents is a good place to store your video. If your electronic medical records include a digital storage file that your family and doctors can access, you can upload the video file there as well. For the technologically savvy, upload a private file to your YouTube channel, Dropbox or another cloud file-hosting service, and give the link to your representative, family and doctors.

• **The more places this file is accessible, the better.** Ensure that your proxy and family won't have to search for your video when it's needed.

• **Update your video as needed.** As with your advance directives in general, you may need to update or change your video if circumstances change in your life that impact your last wishes.

9

Inside a Growing Advocacy

Compassion & Choices has achieved a lot in the last two decades, but the push to create an attitude of empowerment to make choices regarding the end of life has barely taken hold. The path of progress is rarely a graph line in steady ascension. The work often seems slow and grueling. Plenty of setbacks retard progress along the way: betrayals, minor losses, diminished resources and crushing defeats. Our movement has many paladins—those who waged the valiant fight and lost, but advanced the baton nonetheless. And there were many as well who contributed to an eventual victory from which they would never personally benefit.

Most people understand that passing good laws is hard. Elected officials may begin with high ideals and the best interests of their citizens at heart. But even the best intentions often get subverted by a range of forces: pressure to reward campaign donors, professional ambition, personal biases, incomplete knowledge, political opportunities and threats. It's easy to see how the people of the electorate become disillusioned when those they elect fall short of expectations. Indeed, regular people do get short shrift in the halls of government, as the moneyed and corporate interests exert heavy influence day after day.

I awakened to this injustice in 1991, as a newly minted lawyer staffing the Committee on Healthcare and Bioethics in the Oregon State Senate. I remember the moment I first realized the pressing need for citizen activism, especially on behalf of terminally ill

169

people who were powerless and suffering at the end of life. Senator Frank Roberts opened my eyes to this.

Frank Roberts was the most legendary member of the committee. Indeed, he was one of the most distinguished members of the entire legislature. He was a seasoned statesman, so principled and articulate that his colleagues called him the "Conscience of the Senate." His career included many policy achievements, and he also had the distinction of helping to initiate the careers of two early women of prominence in Oregon government. Frank's first wife, Betty, was the first woman to become a justice of the Oregon Supreme Court. His second, Barbara, took office as its first woman governor the same year I joined the senate staff.

Frank became ill with cancer and, by January 1991, it was both advanced and crippling. It was a poignant moment when he watched his wife, Barbara, take the oath of office as governor. Pride and bliss filled his eyes as Barbara leaned down, caressed his face and kissed him. Radiation treatments had injured his spinal cord and he could neither stand nor walk. During the session it was clear that fatigue and pain limited his endurance in prolonged committee hearings. Nevertheless, he was brilliant, keenly astute and physically dashing, even in his decline. He cut a commanding and charismatic figure as he wheeled through the Capitol in a motorized chair.

Frank had introduced death-with-dignity bills in previous legislative sessions, but his colleagues never granted them the slightest consideration. This time it was personal. His own suffering, demise and death stood directly ahead of him, and he wanted a fair hearing for his ideas.

He put his staff to work crafting a well-reasoned bill and started lobbying the committee chairman to allow a full debate. The chairman agreed, but this concession was merely a gesture. The hearing was pure theater. The chairman was giving a nod of respect to a long-serving senator of immense popularity and moral stature, a senator in the throes of a fatal illness. This hearing was a small favor for Frank, nothing more, and certainly not a step on the path to enactment.

On the day of the hearing, the room filled with television crews and newspaper reporters. A cluster of microphones crowded the witness table. A multitude of clergy from many denominations filled the seats. Priests and nuns came decked out in full regalia— stiff habits, robes and headdresses, costumes of doctrinal authority long ago put to rest in closets, only to be retrieved for occasions such as this.

Witnesses supporting the bill were very few. One by one, representatives from churches, hospitals and clinics denounced Frank's bill in the grave tones of dire warning. Surely permitting a dying person to die peacefully in their sleep, with medication prescribed for that purpose, would be an affront to all that is decent and holy, put us on the path to ruin and usher in an apocalypse.

Unheard were the voices of individuals close to the end of their lives, the ones plagued by pain, breathlessness, nausea, seizures and other symptoms that would only worsen as their deadly diseases progressed. Where were the families grieving a loved one who had turned in desperation to a gun, or had leapt from a bridge or balcony to escape unendurable agony? Where were those facing imminent death themselves, to report their terrible fears, not of death, but of the suffering that might precede it? Where were family members who had heard entreaties from loved ones for an ease into death, and who had felt completely helpless and grief-stricken in witness to the suffering of the one they loved? Where were the doctors whose patients had begged them for a merciful gift of medication to end their suffering, who had refused for fear of legal consequences? None of these people were there to tell their stories. So, while Frank's bill did receive a hearing, it never really had a chance.

Frank died in the Governor's Mansion on Halloween night of 1993, having borne exactly the prolonged deterioration and suffering he had hoped to avoid for himself and others. He was a man devoutly faithful to the rule of law. It wasn't in him to obtain aid-in-dying medication and take it surreptitiously. Nor was it in him to use a gun or other violent method to end his life, one that would deepen the grief of those he loved. After he'd been bedridden for weeks, drifting in and out of consciousness, his wife whispered loving words of release into his ear. She understood, she told him, that it was time for her to let him go, that he should "fly like a hawk" and be free.

The very next year a group of advocates gathered in my church. Together, we wrote the Death with Dignity Act. In November 1994, we put it before Oregon voters, who made it the law of the land. Today, a painting of a regal red-tailed hawk adorns my office wall in honor of Senator Frank Roberts.

The Power of Our Stories

My call to advocate for the disempowered and the dying—to grant them autonomy over their suffering and prevent unnecessary tragedies—arrived the day that Frank Roberts' bill died an untimely death before his own passing. I also learned then that the terminally ill will be free of unreasonable restrictions on their end-of-life options only when their stories are heard.

Storytelling remains the first and most effective component of activism. In living rooms and at kitchen tables across the nation, people are telling the stories they have kept in their hearts—stories of loved ones dying, peacefully or with great difficulty. Sometimes the stories are of helping a loved one who begged to die and living with the guilt and shame of having broken the law. And sometimes the stories are of *not* helping one who begged to die, and living with the lingering guilt and shame of abandoning that person in their hour of deepest need.

Stories have the power to cut through political cowardice and legislative obstruction. Keeping silent only perpetuates the injustice enacted by establishment gatekeepers and lawmakers bound to old biases. Telling our stories can turn lawmakers to the task of serving the people they represent. The dying, the suffering and the witnesses to senseless agony must be silent no more.

Oregon was the pioneer that carved a path in the wilderness and cleared the ground that every other state in the nation might

How to Become a Storyteller

Poignant end-of-life stories like that of Brittany Maynard can inspire people to action in ways that data or statistics cannot.

Compassion & Choices collects stories and personal experiences from people across the nation and puts them to work to change minds and hearts and inform public policy. Yours could be the story that inspires the next leap in the movement for end-of-life choices.

People with advancing illnesses can tell their stories of exercising discernment in choosing treatment options, to help break the cycle of "conveyor belt" healthcare. Family members who have seen the impact of having choices on the quality of a loved one's life have important information to share. Those who have borne witness to a difficult death, with few options, also have a powerful story to tell.

Compassion & Choices' Storyteller Program captures, on video or through other media, the powerful personal stories of those who have shared in the end-of-life experience. If you believe you have a story that could benefit the end-of-life care movement, please contact the Storyteller Program at CompassionAndChoices.org/stories.

A few tips for crafting your story are outlined below:

• Review the main discussion points around current end-of-life issues and look at your own experience to see how it adds to the discussion.

• The best stories in support of a cause have a clear point. What is the one-line "headline" for your story?

• Names and personal details help a story feel real.

• Look for specific moments that illustrate the issue or that were a turning point and describe them in personal terms.

• How does what's happening/already happened make you feel? Sharing your feelings triggers empathy in listeners, which helps them understand and identify with the issue.

• Look for instances of cause and effect. These helps persuade listeners and make clear the reality of a situation.

• End with a call for action. What do you hope listeners will be compelled to do after hearing your story?

traverse. Not far to the north, a great man was watching. Having spent an illustrious career in politics, Booth Gardner, former governor of the state of Washington, was well aware of medical aid in dying as a political issue. But it didn't mean much to him until he himself experienced the symptoms and anxieties of Parkinson's disease. It changed his life to experience his body becoming weak and unreliable. Suddenly, he had his own story to tell.

"I've got a lot of things going on in my mind these days because life hasn't gone the way I planned it," he told an interviewer during this time. "And I have to be honest with you. Not a day goes by that I don't think about death now. When I wake up and I'm getting ready to go out of the house, I kid myself: I say, is this the day? Is this where you're going to be found in the bathroom? I don't want that, so I take short showers these days. I just get in and get out, and I'm out of there. There's more times I've forgotten to rinse my head than I want to tell you."

Booth was the governor of Washington from 1985 to 1993, and his popularity was legend. Midway through his tenure, he won re-election by the most dramatic landslide victory of any modern governor. Despite, or because of, a difficult beginning in life, the desire to help people drove his work, and his authentic concern for others was unmistakable.

Booth's early life was one of material privilege and emotional hardship. At age four, he played the unwilling pawn in his parents' bitter and very public divorce. His father, who won custody, was an angry alcoholic. When Booth was 14, his mother and sister died in a plane crash. And when he was barely into his twenties, his father jumped or fell to his death from a hotel balcony in Honolulu. During his college years, Booth worked as a coach and tutor to local kids in the largely African-American central district of the Washington Parks Department. This experience was both formative and transformative.

"Prejudice just went right over my head," he recalled. "I saw kids with severe disabilities and met their brave and frustrated parents ... even though I thought I'd been pretty much hammered

... they had it a lot worse ... I settled down in school and started to work hard because I realized I couldn't get to my goal if I didn't get out of college. I wanted to make a difference."

And make a difference he did. During his time in office, Gardner championed—and signed into law—a program in which health care for the working poor would be covered by state medical insurance. He dramatically increased spending on early childhood education and state universities. He was a tireless champion of the environment. He appointed the first minority to the State Supreme Court, an African-American man named Charles Z. Smith. Booth recognized Native tribal sovereignty and strengthened legal protections for gay people.

His constituents were shocked when he didn't seek a third term. Unbeknownst even to him, Parkinson's was already ravaging his system. All he knew at that point was that his energy level was not what it had been, and in his heart, he felt he was not up to what the position demanded and deserved. A year after leaving office, Booth received the official diagnosis of Parkinson's disease.

Fifteen years later, in a documentary about his last political campaign, he would tell the interviewer: "My quality of life today is okay because I can still function, but I can feel daily little things that are different. Like I slur a little bit when I talk. I've had walking problems lately. Your walking and your voice go. Then your ability to eat goes. And when you can't eat or keep anything down, you starve to death. And it's not a pretty picture.

"I automatically thought I had control over the rest of my life. It never dawned on me that I don't have any control. But that's the fact. I think that's wrong."

Early in 2006, Booth was in Olympia receiving an award for his public service and, as he was leaving the stage, an audience member yelled, "What are you going to do next?" Booth returned to the microphone to address the question.

"This is not going to sit well with some of you, I'm afraid, but I just want to be honest and straightforward with you," he said from the stage. "I've made all the tough decisions in my life: where

I wanted to go to college, who I wanted to marry, how many kids I wanted to have. Those were all critical decisions in my life and I made them myself. And I think I ought to have the right to make the last decision: when it's time for me to go, and how I go. So, I'm going to head up an initiative and we're going to get that assisted death in this state."

There was a hushed pause in which the audience seemed to be startled into silence. But perhaps no one was more surprised than Booth when, a moment later, they rose almost as one in a standing ovation.

Before Booth emerged on the scene, we at Compassion & Choices were already talking with our affiliate in the state of Washington about what it would take to launch a campaign in that state. We conducted polling and focus groups and had several brainstorming sessions. We had begun to craft a proposed law, but funding a campaign was our major concern. At that point, we didn't know about Booth's intentions and thought we were the logical campaign organizers. We were veterans of two successful campaigns and had spent three intense years defending Oregon's Death with Dignity law from a slew of legal opponents. Twice we had brought the argument all the way to the U.S. Supreme Court. We felt seasoned and successful.

Then we learned that Booth shared our goal. On February 24, 2006, I traveled to Seattle to have lunch with Booth at the Compassion & Choices regional office located there. Booth had not yet received the treatment that would later reverse some of his Parkinson's symptoms and it was sometimes difficult to understand his speech. Nevertheless, he projected unwavering confidence and abiding good nature. He looked at us, the supposed "experts" seated around the table. Then he jabbed his thumb back over his shoulder and said, with absolute authority, "We're going to have a campaign, and I want you all to get in line behind me." So, we did.

The next month we began to formalize the coalition behind the 2008 Washington "I-1000" ballot initiative. Four organizations, Compassion & Choices, Compassion & Choices of Washington, Death with Dignity National Center and Booth's political action committee, called *Dignity 2007*, met regularly at a location midway between Portland and Seattle. Dr. Tom Preston, retired Seattle cardiologist and early activist with Compassion in Dying (a predecessor organization to Compassion & Choices), served as the central organizer and mediator. He steered us through robust dialogue and debate around the language of the bill and the structure of the campaign. It was during these meetings that we determined the essential elements of the bill and made plans to raise the $3.5 to $5.2 million needed to win.

Also, in these meetings, it was with some frustration and sadness that Booth realized he would probably never qualify to benefit personally from the law he was working so hard to pass. Because of the chronic and unpredictable nature of Parkinson's disease, doctors find it difficult to predict when people with Parkinson's disease are likely to die, thus prohibiting them from having the end-of-life choices given to people who will die within six months.

In early 2008, we were ready to go, and Booth filed a medical aid in dying initiative with the Washington Secretary of State. A month later, the campaign was well underway and known as *Yes on I-1000*. Compassion & Choices of Washington threw all the passion and dedication of its staff and volunteers into the campaign. They recruited and trained a team of over 1,000 volunteers, who fanned out over the state to collect signatures to place the initiative on the November ballot. They helped recruit storytellers and gained endorsements from many community and seniors organizations. They manned booths at church events and county fairs. Everyone's combined efforts yielded almost 100,000 signatures more than what was required to get the initiative on the ballot.

Booth was tireless and generous. He gave $300,000 out of his own pocket to the campaign, making him its largest single donor. During this time, he also made many appearances in the media. In his 2009 documentary, he testified about the many citizens in need of this law. "I hear a story a day," he said. "I can't get away from stories of people who are in deep suffering and that gets me a little angry, but it makes me believe I've got to see this thing through."

In another interview, Booth spun a poignantly simple fantasy of the death he wanted. He explained, "I think about it being a Sunday afternoon: summertime, nice day. My grandkids are around. I've got eight of them. My wife is there, and I call everybody together and I say, I'm not getting any better. I've had a great life. Next Friday, I want to end it. Let's spend this week saying goodbye to each other."

When asked for his response to the objections cited by the proposed law's opponents in the church, Booth reflected that many such people had told him that God had His own plan for the end of his life. And then he said, "I don't believe God has any kind of plan that causes me to suffer in the latter years of my life. I've served Him well. I was put on the earth with a certain set of skills, I was told to go out and do the best I can with what I was given ... and along the way, help others if I could. You're going to get blindsided, you're going to have things happen that you don't understand, but keep going, you can have a good life.

"And I've had a good life. I had a lousy childhood, so I've come out of a rough spot and made a good life for myself. I want folks to be able to go out with dignity."

Much of the campaign played out in the media, with dueling spokespeople speaking from their own perspective. A woman named Nancy Niedzielski played a central role, talking about her husband Randy's death from brain cancer, and her promise to him to make assistance in dying a legal option. She overcame her own shyness to come forward and stand before microphones and cameras, audiences and interviewers, again and again. Often bringing her audience to tears, she unabashedly asked them straight out, "Please help me keep my promise to my husband."

The actor Martin Sheen shot an opposition ad. He told viewers from behind a presidential-looking desk that I-1000 was a dangerous policy and would hurt vulnerable people. On our side, Barbara Roberts, former governor of Oregon, appeared as the ultimate validator, vouching for the safety and popularity of Oregon's Death with Dignity law.

On election night, we gathered at the Rock Bottom Brewery in downtown Seattle to watch returns come in. Almost 3 million people voted on the initiative, nearly 58 percent in favor and about 42 percent in opposition. It was a wide margin, and a ringing endorsement of Booth and his honest intention to bring peace and comfort to dying people.

Facing the TV cameras at the brewery that night, Booth offered this poignant statement:

> "On election night I do not allow myself to get too happy. For every high there is a corresponding low, and when elected governor twice I knew much work lay ahead. But I am exceptionally happy tonight. The difference? We the people have made law together in a shared undertaking, and on this at least our work is done ... So, thank you again, each of you, and thanks to our blessed democratic process and the wondrous will of the people."

Like Frank Roberts, however, Booth would, in the end, die unassisted by the very right he worked so hard to achieve for others. Still, it was his condition that had made him intimately aware of the need for this legislation. A public servant to the end, he spent his precious remaining time in the service of something far vaster than himself.

Montana's "Regular Guy"

The luminaries of our victories haven't always been public figures.

If Frank Robert's counterpart in Washington was a seasoned statesman like himself, his counterpart in Montana was the opposite. A former U.S. Marine, long-haul trucker and avid outdoorsman, Robert Baxter was very much a "regular guy." After enduring a dozen years of cancer treatment for lymphocytic leukemia, Baxter chose to discontinue chemotherapy at the age of 76.

Before long, he had dwindled to skeletal proportions. "He was so skinny he couldn't sit because his skin hurt," his daughter Roberta reflected afterwards. "It pinched his skin together because there was no meat. It was that bad."

Baxter decided he wanted to hasten the end of his life, but no doctor would write him the requisite prescription. So, in 2008, he sought out Mark Connell, a local attorney.

"Bob approached us and asked if there was anything we could do from a legal standpoint to try to gain access to medications that, if he chose to use them, would hasten his death," said Connell. "He knew he was going to die, the only question was how long that was going to take and how much suffering he was going to go through."

If Baxter was a departure from the previous two statesmen, Montana itself was also a departure from the emerging pattern. Until then, medical aid in dying had generally presented as a progressive issue. Washington and Oregon are two of the bluest states in the union. Montana, on the other hand, has long been the domain of conservative Republicans. But in the full circle of politics, there are places where the left and the right meet in agreement, and Montana proved to be one such place. "There's a long tradition here going back to frontier days of people basically saying that there are certain areas the government ought to stay out of," said Connell.

Baxter felt much the same way. "The lawsuit was one of the things my father was passionate about in the end," his daughter Roberta recalled. "He wanted to stay alive to get it done."

When Connell won the case before a district judge, he called Baxter to share the news. "His wife answered the phone," Connell recalled. "I told her what had happened and she said, 'Well, Bob would be delighted,' but he was asleep right then and not available to come to the phone. And the irony is, he never woke up. Bob died December 5, 2008, without ever learning he'd just won that case."

When the verdict was later appealed, Baxter's daughter took up the torch of his advocacy, presenting statements to the Montana Supreme Court on his behalf. Compassion & Choices helped in the litigation of that case, and dozens of Montana state legislators and human rights groups filed briefs as "friends of the court." The state's Supreme Court ruled that nothing in state law made medical aid in dying illegal, and that it did not violate public policy. Still, the fight was not over.

Within a few years, State Representative Krayton Kearns began a campaign to introduce bills to overturn the Supreme Court ruling. "Our lives do in effect belong to God," he told an interviewer for Reason TV. "He will call us when it's time and not before. It's the way I live my life and the way I would encourage other people to live theirs."

When asked whether he thought it appropriate for religion to be injected into politics, Krayton replied, "Without a doubt. Without a doubt. Because we cannot separate the two."

On the opposite side was Dr. Eric Kress, a Missoula physician with a family practice. He never set out to be at the forefront of the controversy, but his experience with a terminal patient changed everything.

"He was a man who was now 120 pounds of skin and bone," Dr. Kress recalled. "He used to be over 6'2" and he had been a very strong, physical, athletic man. He made his desire and intentions very well known to me: that he wanted this medication. But it was new, I wasn't all that familiar with it, and he became very angry with me. He dressed me down, he yelled at me. He also called me a coward. He made me think about this situation.

"And what happened is I didn't write him the prescription and then within a month or two he had stockpiled enough medication. He ingested a large amount and ended up killing himself. And I had to kind of ask myself, you know: *Why didn't I do it? I can do this. Am I worried about me, or am I going to worry about him?*"

Subsequently, Dr. Kress became an outspoken advocate for medical aid in dying. In his testimony before the Senate Judiciary

Committee during the hearing for the Kearns bill, he said, "This bill clearly states that any doctor, nurse or family member who assists a patient in obtaining an aid-in-dying prescription will be sentenced to ten years in prison and fined $50,000. So, you may be wondering, what kind of doctor is it that you will be sending to jail? I stand before you today and state that I am that kind of doctor. I have written an aid-in-dying prescription on three occasions."

I have rarely witnessed such a public display of courage.

Dr. Kress concluded, "I urge you to vote against House Bill 505, a bill that would be the government taking a personal freedom that the citizens of Montana now enjoy."

In a later comment on the controversy, he said, "We do have a tradition in the U.S. that the government really doesn't get in the way of the doctor and the patient and their decision-making [about] what's right for them. Especially [regarding] what a doctor and a patient would talk about. We're supposed to have free speech and you're telling me what I can or can't talk to a patient about? That is crazy. This is not good for America, for Montana, or patients and doctors."

The Kearns bill to overturn the Supreme Court ruling failed in the Montana Senate, and every similar bill in subsequent legislative sessions has also failed. Medical aid in dying remains legal in Montana today.

Heroes Who Advanced Our Nation's Dialogue and Understanding

Finally, as I mentioned earlier, heroes of our movement include those who persisted, but did not prevail. Nevertheless, these people advanced our nation's dialogue and understanding, kept the conversation going about a taboo subject and helped bend the long arc of human history toward justice.

The most recognizable face of California's multi-year campaign for medical aid in dying will always be Brittany Maynard. It was her prophetic voice that finally cracked the political logjam in Sacramento. And though our gratitude to Brittany cannot be overstated, our movement owes as much to the unsung civil servants, such as the tireless campaigner, Former California State Assemblywoman Patty Berg. Not long ago, a young Compassion & Choices volunteer interviewed Berg for our archives. Though I knew her story well and had lived it with her, it was still moving to hear her tell it. Patty worked from every imaginable angle for years to advance medical aid in dying in the California legislature.

No one can tell her story with more accuracy and immediacy than Patty herself, and her words reveal how extraordinarily difficult it is to enact a law that is supported by the people but opposed by entrenched political operatives. Here, in Patty's own words, are insights into the rough and tumble of politics and the competition of forces on opposite sides.

> I carried the bill three times. I started in 2005 and I had a co-author named Lloyd Levine. He had a grandparent who had died tragically of cancer and he was passionate about the issue. I was passionate about the issue too and had been for a long time. I'd worked in the field of aging for 20 years before I ran for the state legislature.
>
> I knew I wanted to carry this bill when I was elected in 2002. When you work in the field of aging, you have sympathy cards on your desk all the time. I had known several people who'd died of terrible cancers, in pain and begging for relief. I'd also lost my husband to a massive stroke. Had he survived it, I know he would have been begging me to help him, too. And as a physician, he would have assisted such patients if they asked. I know he would have.
>
> So, it was a professional thing but also a personal thing for me. And it was something that I would want for myself. My whole stance was that it was about choice,

it was about protecting privacy, it was about civil rights, and it was about separation of church and state. That was part of the message we consistently delivered.

So, in 2005, we introduced Bill AB 654. Before we introduced the bill, we decided to hold two informational hearings, one in Los Angeles and one in Sacramento. We really brought a lot of people into the discussion and had fabulous speakers.

In 2005, it got as far as the Assembly Judiciary Committee. To get it out of the Assembly, you needed 41 votes. I had 14 co-authors on the bill, but the sponsor decided we should hold it on the floor because there was no way I was going to be able to get 41 votes. I had personal meetings with every single one of the 120 legislators. I sat down with every Republican and every Democrat, telling them why it was so important to me. We didn't have a single Republican vote for any of the three bills. And we had vehement opposition every step of the way from the California Medical Association and the Roman Catholic Church. The church targeted the Latinos in the legislature, of which there were quite a few, threatening that they could not receive communion if they supported this.

The Latinos were all Roman Catholics and many of them had mothers who had come from Mexico and they were very family-oriented. And yet these Latinos were all Democrats who were pro-choice regarding abortion, because you simply cannot get elected as a Democrat in California unless you're pro-choice. And what sense does it make to be pro-choice at the beginning of life and not at the end? That was part of my argument.

Now abortion, medical aid in dying and marriage equality were the major issues of the Catholic church. Every

Latino was pro-choice and, in being so, had likely gone against their parents and grandparents with regard to reproduction. And we had carried the marriage equality bill in California too. So, it was almost as if there was this rule: you can go against your family once or twice, but you can't do it three times.

During this time, I also got a letter from my bishop. This was the diocese of Santa Rosa, so he oversaw all the parishes in Northern California, from Sonoma County all the way to the Oregon border, including mine. There was an article in The San Francisco Chronicle about this bill, because it was covered in every major newspaper in the state. And just as an aside, all the major newspapers in the state endorsed this bill—they all supported it.

Anyway, this article identified me as a Roman Catholic carrying this bill. So, I get a letter from Bishop Daniel Walsh:

"I'm writing today because of the article that appeared in the January 2 SF Chronicle about your sponsorship of a bill allowing physician-assisted suicide. In the article, you were quoted as saying: "I am a Roman Catholic." This statement has caused a scandal among the Catholic community. The church has enunciated the natural law against suicide by citing the fifth commandment: thou shalt not kill. And it has taught throughout its history that life is a gift from God that must be protected and supported. The catechism of the Catholic Church treats the matter of suicide very directly ...

You assert that you are a Catholic and the same time you sponsor a bill that is contrary to the teachings of the Church which is founded in the natural law and the commandments. This is troubling to me as well as the Catholic community. In my role of bishop and teacher of the faith in the diocese of Santa Rosa, I have concern that the faithful not be confused on what the church teaches and that you understand the position of the church in this matter. Again, I ask to have a chance to speak with you in a private manner so that we can understand each other in the situation."

So, of course, I called to set up a meeting. And he met with me along with another priest who was an attorney for the diocese. I think we probably met for two hours in my office in Sacramento at the capitol. I thought I was going to be threatened with excommunication. My name was being spoken from the pulpit in churches throughout California because the church ran its own campaign against this bill. They were handing out post-cards at every mass, they were preaching against it in their Sunday sermons, the priests were reading letters from this bishop to their congregants. And my name was invoked continually. It was horrible.

So, I met with the bishop and his attorney and I said, "We obviously disagree on this issue and I'm hoping we can disagree without being disagreeable." And I went into why I was fighting for this piece of legislation and why I thought it was important and we talked about it. But right before we completed the meeting, I said I knew that as the bishop of this diocese, he would be issuing a letter on the subject to all his parishes. 'But,' I told him, 'I would caution you not to use the word *scandal* in your letter. And I say that because two priests from my parish [St. Joseph's] are both serving prison time for violating young boys. Two other priests in our county'—of course he knew all of this—'committed violent suicide because they were accused of molesting young boys. And the bishop that preceded you was having an affair with a priest in Ukiah who was stealing money from the church! So, I would caution you not to use the word *scandal*.'

After our meeting, he sent me a letter saying he appreciated my time and he thought it was advantageous to have met with me personally. He said he would be writing to his people concerning this matter. And he enclosed a copy of the letter. It did not include the word *scandal*.

Cracking the California Medical Association (CMA) was the real issue. And one of my good friends, Luther Cobb, was very politically active within the CMA. The CMA has something called the House of Delegates, and every year they have a gathering of members who are elected to represent their local medical societies, and that is called their House of Delegates meeting. And they take positions on various issues. We knew we had to get a resolution into the House of Delegates for the CMA to consider changing its position in opposition to this bill. They'd opposed medical aid in dying all along on the grounds that they're healers, not killers. So, we got Luther to carry a resolution into that annual meeting, a resolution that they would support the pending medical aid in dying bill. It was voted down unanimously, but at least we got it introduced as a resolution. It was just one more piece of strategy. You can't imagine how time-consuming this bill was. We had so many press conferences. We were trying to defend it from every angle. Ultimately it was decided that we would park the bill and not carry it forward because we clearly weren't going to get the votes needed to pass it.

Then in 2006, we decided we were going to bring it back, this time starting in the Senate. Lloyd and I thought we might have a better chance there because the Senate was a little more liberal. So, we decided we would substitute the language in a pending Senate bill and make that bill the medical aid-in-dying bill.

The story of this bill is the Joe Dunn story. Joe Dunn was a senator. He chaired the Judiciary Committee on the Senate side and you always meet with the Chair of the Committee first. Because more often than not, members of the same party will vote with the Chair. It's just the way it works. So, Joe Dunn had always been a fairly progressive senator, he'd been in the legislature a long time, he was well regarded, well thought-of, and I had a good relationship with him.

He basically made me a promise that he would be in support of the bill. And then he started toying around and told me at one point that he wanted to have a separate hearing on the bill before it was considered by the committee. So, we arranged for an information hearing a week before the bill was scheduled to be up before his committee.

Now every committee has standing consultants that work with it. And his chief consultant was a guy who was known as the 41st Senator. He was vehemently opposed to the bill, and the bill analysis that came out of the Senate Judiciary Committee was the most negative bill analysis that I have ever read.

We held the informational hearing and many wonderful people came to testify: physicians and ethicists, people who had experienced cancer. So, after essentially committing to me that he was going to vote 'Aye,' we had the meeting the following week and he spoke for 15 minutes and then he voted 'No.' And every other Democrat voted 'Yes.' He betrayed me. It was his last year in the Senate and he lined up with the CMA when he cast that deciding vote. He killed the bill when he could have legalized it, could have moved it. Well, wouldn't you know what happened next? The following year, he was termed out of the Senate and he was hired as the CEO of the CMA. It was a terrible double-cross.

The third time around, in 2007, we decided we were going to offer the bill as Assembly Bill 374. Fabian Nunez—a Latino—was the Speaker of the Assembly, which is the most powerful position within that body, and I asked him to be a joint author on the bill. After that, it wasn't just Lloyd and Patty anymore, it was the Speaker. And he was just great. He said, "Oh my God, my mother is just going to go crazy." And he also had to endure the Cardinal—Cardinal Roger Mahoney— attacking him at a mass, saying that he supported the culture of death. It was horrible.

I had 27 co-authors on AB 374 and I had the Speaker as a joint author and that's a lot. I had 35 committed votes. We got it through the Judiciary Committee, we got it through Appropriations committee. I had 35 'Ayes' but I was 6 short which was too many for the Speaker to have to work. It's too many. Three is okay, but not six. I had at least four people tell me, 'I'll be the 41st vote, Patty, but I'm not going to be the 36th vote.' I'll tell you, it takes guts to do some of these things. This was the most controversial bill in the legislature all three years. The most controversial. More so than marriage equality. And people kept being threatened by their church. People had their various excuses.

Anyway, we got it to the floor. Lloyd and I really wanted a debate on the floor but ultimately it was decided that course was too risky. The risk was a third public defeat. That was the bottom line. I was disappointed, really disappointed that we couldn't have the debate. But we chose to hold it on the floor, which means the bill would not pass.

Ultimately, eight years later, the game-changer was Brittany Maynard. Finally, the timing was just right. The End of Life Option Act of 2015 had two great authors in the Senate, Bill Monning and Lois Wolk, both of whom I served with, both wonderful people. Susan Eggman carried the bill in the Assembly; she had a PhD in social work and she'd worked at a hospice in Oregon. I was retired by then but worked behind the scenes to help get 50 state legislators to sign on as co-authors. And I was instrumental in getting the CMA to withdraw its long-standing opposition and be neutral. Remember Luther Cobb? Well, Luther was the president of the CMA that year. California was the first medical society in the country to vote to be neutral on the issue and their neutrality was absolutely vital.

In October 2015, when Governor Jerry Brown of California signed the bill into law, the white-hot spotlight of victory was not trained on Patty Berg. But her contributions were undeniable and indispensable.

The Disconnect Between the People and the Politicians

As Patty's decade-long story demonstrates, most politicians remain unwilling to buck political power houses like organized religion and organized medicine to vote for medical aid in dying. For over 20 years, in legislature after legislature, bills have been introduced, but victories have been mostly elusive. Only Vermont, California, Hawai'i, Maine and New Jersey have succeeded in passing these bills, and this happened only after 20 years of concerted effort in Hawai'i and over ten each in Vermont, Maine and

California and seven years in New Jersey.

Opponents portray these long struggles as proof that medical aid in dying is unpopular. But that is not so. The truth is that it's very hard to get bills passed through any legislative body. The system strongly favors the status quo and politicians usually see inaction as the safest route to reelection. Medical aid in dying is a policy that has always had enormous public support but must overcome the combined forces of inertia and strong opposition from a powerful minority in state legislatures. Recent polls by Gallup and Harris show 69 to 74 percent of people believe terminally ill adults should have access to medical means to bring about a peaceful death. This belief is strong throughout the nation and across all demographic categories, including age, disability, religion and political party.

The disconnect between the people and elected politicians is beginning to resolve, for several reasons.

First, in 2014, Brittany Maynard succeeded in communicating the urgency that dying people feel—when unbearable suffering looms upon them and they simply cannot wait another 20 years for politicians to heed their pleas.

Second, claims of harm to vulnerable people and to the institution of medicine simply do not hold up in the face of overwhelming evidence to the contrary. Between Oregon, Washington, Montana, Vermont, California, Colorado and Washington, D.C., we now have 40 years of combined experience with authorized medical aid in dying. Within all that data, there is not one episode of abuse, coercion or participation of an unqualified individual.

Increasingly, lawmakers who vote down medical aid in dying by voicing vague concerns, unsubstantiated threats and unspecified risks do not appear thoughtful or reasonable. They just seem cruel.

Third, with the authorizing of medical aid in dying in New Jersey in 2019, over 20 percent of the U.S. population has this right. Increasingly, people in these states will experience the peace of mind and improved quality of life brought by the choice of medical aid in dying to those with terminal illness. Stories of these benefits will pass from state to state via relatives, friends, professional networks and educational forums. Soon, the weight of knowledge and experience will discredit the hyperbolic stories and hypothetical dangers that have so often swayed legislative bodies in the past.

The American legislative process failed Frank Roberts and many like him, but it will not fail the rest of us forever. Baby boomers have seen their parents die hard deaths, and they are vowing it

Your First Steps to Advocacy

If you want to act on your support for the exploding movement to improve the end-of-life experience, volunteering with Compassion & Choices (C&C), the nation's oldest, largest and most active nonprofit organization working to improve care and expand options for the end of life, can be rewarding and highly effective. For more than 30 years, C&C has recruited, trained and deployed volunteers for social change. C&C offers plenty of support and meaningful opportunities to new advocates.

Below are some of the actions you might take in your first steps to advocacy. (More info about the actions below can be found at CompassionAndChoices.org/volunteer.)

• Join a Volunteer Action Team in your region. Over 7,000 volunteers work in 100 action teams throughout the nation. You may also start an Action Team if there is none in your area.

• Work with your state's team leaders to craft a letter to the editor of your local newspaper about your thoughts on end-of-life issues. Include reasons you support the expansion of options to include medical aid in dying.

• Sign up for email bulletins on advocacy opportunities taking place near you.

• Volunteer to participate in an informational phone bank (from will be different for the ones they love and for themselves. Young people are educated, energized and joining a movement they once thought did not concern them. Healthcare consumers are applying the primary lessons of the natural birthing and AIDS movements to the movement for end-of-life rights: that the fight to empower patients must start with them.

home) or staff the C&C booth at a local fair or event, talking with visitors and handing out literature.

• Participate in Ask Your Doctor and/or Ask Your Candidate campaigns by making a point to ask your doctors and political candidates if they support the medical aid-in-dying option and share with them why you support it.

• Communicate with your political representatives, either in their local offices or in their state legislative offices, to show your support for expanded options at the end of life.

• Carry a C&C petition to local events and ask people who support medical aid in dying to add their names.

• Ask other groups you belong to if they would host a presentation on end-of-life issues or the medical aid-in-dying option, specifically.

• Hold a screening of the documentary film *How to Die in Oregon* in your home or at a local community space, like a library or senior center. If a copy of the film is unavailable at your local library, you can order it by emailing clearcutfilms@gmail.com.

• Browse the Volunteer Brownbag Archives at CompassionAndChoices. org/volunteer. These include compelling, hour-long recorded sessions with leaders of the medical aid-in-dying movement.

Few of these excellent first steps to advocacy take a lot of time. Find out more at CompassionAndChoices.org/volunteer.

10

People Taking Control

As we've seen, our culture often pushes us to pursue treatments to fight a disease at any cost. We've looked at the many ways the deck is stacked against deciding to lead a full life as illness advances and opting for a peaceful death. We've learned that arranging a peaceful death that serves your values and priorities can be accomplished in a number of ways: by deciding to stop eating and drinking, by stopping life-sustaining treatment like kidney dialysis or by abbreviating the dying process through terminal sedation or medical aid in dying in those states that authorize this.

Obstacles may arise both inside and outside of the medical establishment. Some of these obstacles are legal, some are religious, some are social and some are emotional. The stories in this chapter show just a few of the ways these obstacles, and the forces behind them, can wreak havoc on the best-laid plans we've made to honor our values and priorities in life's final chapter. The stories also show how some people have managed to navigate this obstacle course successfully and fulfill their dying wishes.

Overcoming Roadblocks to a Peaceful Death

In February 2013, Barbara Mancini's father, Joe Yourshaw, was dying of diabetes, kidney failure and heart problems in the little town of Pottsville, Pennsylvania. Joe had already enrolled in hospice care at home, where he planned to die peacefully. It was noted in his hospice record that he was "adamant" that he never wanted to go to the hospital. He had taken all the conscientious measures that someone at the end of life could take. He had completed his advance directive. He had signed a Do Not Resuscitate order. His loved ones were well aware of his wishes. And he had designated his daughter Barbara, a registered nurse, as his healthcare proxy. Everything was in place to ensure a tranquil death at home.

What happened, however, could not have been further from the end Joe intended.

This 93-year-old man, in the throes of multiple organ failure, was experiencing many of the escalating symptoms common to those in their final days. Pain was one of these symptoms and shortness of breath was another.

Barbara had traveled to be at his bedside and during the worst pain he had ever experienced to that point, Joe asked Barbara to hand him his 1-ounce vial of morphine.

She passed him the vial and was startled when he drank it all.

"Gee, Dad," she said, "that's a lot of morphine." But given the fact that he was 93 years old, actively dying and in considerable pain, it never occurred to her to treat this turn of events as some kind of medical emergency.

Soon afterward, Joe's hospice nurse arrived and found him drowsy, but able to follow commands and respond to questions. Without prompting, Barbara voluntarily told the hospice nurse that her father, without warning, had taken a large dose of morphine.

The nurse called her supervisor, who called the police. Within the hour, Joe was in the hospital—the last place he'd wanted to be—and subjected to a morphine antidote.

And to make a preposterous situation still more surreal, his beloved daughter was under arrest.

When Joe regained consciousness, it would be impossible to overstate how distressed he was to learn that Barbara was in police custody. Against his will, Joe was kept in the hospital (where, of course, he was given more morphine, since he was in undeniable pain and dying). He lingered this way the last five days of his life, after which the coroner pronounced his death a homicide.

Barbara was formally charged with aiding an attempted suicide. Compassion & Choices was called in to advise her legal team and publicize her case. Dozens of opinion writers across the nation weighed in on the injustice of charging Barbara with this felony and attempting to impose the penalty of ten years in prison.

But the prosecution effort would not be daunted. Schuylkill County District Attorney Karen Noone, who was appointed to her office and was running in her first election to retain her position, handed off the case to Pennsylvania Attorney General Kathleen Kane's office. Noone said she made this decision because her friendship with Barbara's younger sister created a conflict of interest. Kane's office decided to prosecute the case aggressively.

It took a full year from the time of Barbara's arrest until her case was dismissed. The state court's opinion vindicated her; it stated that the case against her was based on nothing but hearsay and conjecture and should not have been brought in the first place. The attorney general decided not to appeal.

But the damage was done. Joe's death had been deeply traumatic, and the aftermath for his daughter was more traumatic still. Barbara lost a year fighting the charges against her and incurred legal fees exceeding $100,000. During this time, she'd been suspended from her job as a nurse and was unable to earn an income, while her husband was forced to work double shifts as a paramedic to make ends meet. Compassion & Choices set up a fund to help defray the legal fees but there was no way to offset the emotional cost.

I believe prosecutors pursue charges like this one to make an example of people like Barbara. They hope cases like hers will serve as a deterrent to every person at the bedside of a dying loved one. And they do. The fear instilled guarantees that many families will ignore their loved ones' pleas and desperate patients will die with profound suffering, or violently and alone.

Diane Rehm's Heartfelt Connection to the Issue

A powerful critic of the legal roadblocks to a peaceful death is prominent radio host Diane Rehm, of National Public Radio (NPR).

Diane has a personal reason for adding her voice to the struggle. She had a longtime pact with John, her husband of 55 years, that they would help each other die if that time should arrive.

For John, that time came when Parkinson's disease so ravaged him that he no longer had the use of his hands—no longer had the ability to feed himself, bathe or engage in any activity. He pleaded with his physician for medication to help him die but the doctor refused, because assistance was illegal in Maryland. Diane was pointedly warned not to help him either.

I think it's important to note here that most commentators do believe it is criminal to assist someone in dying, or for a doctor to respond to a request from a terminally ill, mentally competent patient and provide medication the patient could take themselves to die peacefully, except in states where medical aid in dying is specifically authorized.

But whether this conduct qualifies as the crime of assisting (that is, aiding and abetting) a suicide, in states where medical aid in dying is not authorized is not so clear. A study published in the *New England Journal of Medicine* in 1996 found that 20 percent of physicians surveyed had knowingly and intentionally prescribed medication to hasten a patient's death. That's a very large percentage, yet to my knowledge, no physician in any state has ever been prosecuted for providing medication for peaceful dying to a qualified patient.

Dr. Timothy Quill came the closest to being prosecuted when in 1991 he reported in the *New England Journal of Medicine* that he had given Diane, a patient dying of leukemia, a prescription for medication which she subsequently took and then died peacefully. Dr. Quill did not intend to challenge the law. He intended to advance the compassionate practice of medicine. The New York Attorney General saw it differently and brought the doctor before a grand jury. After hearing the evidence, the jury declined to indict Dr. Quill for assisting a suicide or for any other crime.

Litigation can help clarify the law, and Compassion & Choices succeeded in removing some of the confusion over medical aid in dying in Montana, when that state's supreme court found, in Baxter v. Montana, that there was no clear legislative ban against it and no conflict with public policy. Doctors have practiced medical aid in dying openly in Montana since 2009. In 2019, C&C has a similar lawsuit underway in Massachusetts. Some states, like Idaho and Georgia, have responded to the ambiguity by specifically making it illegal to prescribe medication intended to cause death. But the law remains murky in many states, including Maryland.

Murky or not, given the common assumption about doctors being at risk of criminal prosecution, it seemed only one avenue was available for John Rehm to advance the time of his death: voluntarily stopping all food and fluids. So, he resolved not to eat or drink. It took John ten long days to die. Rehm felt the way her husband had to die was cruel, inexcusable and just plain wrong.

Because of her heartfelt connection to this issue, Rehm has since conducted a series of interviews highlighting not only the legal barriers to dying well, but many of the social and emotional ones as well.

One such conversation was with Dr. Kathleen Morris, a physician in Oregon, the state that passed the original Death with Dignity Act in 1997. Morris had written a medical aid-in-dying prescription at the request of her patient, Cody Curtis, who was dying of liver cancer. Dr. Morris readily admitted that this had not been easy for her to do. In their interview, Rehm asked her how she had come to the decision to provide medical aid in dying as a doctor—and how she reconciled that choice with the well-known admonition that physicians must do no harm.

Morris revealed that to write the prescription, she had to confront her own grief—a confrontation many doctors will do anything to avoid. "I think I struggled with the decision because I wanted so desperately to continue to have Cody in my life and in the lives of her family and friends ... She was a remarkable human being and just ... a wonderful source of life and light on this planet," she told Rehm. "And yet ... I knew she was going to face a pretty ugly end, and that would have been hard for her as a very dignified person."

Morris confided next that Cody gave her time to think it over. She understood the emotional stakes were high and she told her doctor she'd understand if it were too difficult. But Cody was clear this option was what she wanted to access. Morris spent the next several days talking with her family and friends about Cody's request and she decided that, as her physician, it was the right thing to do.

Regarding the part of the Hippocratic Oath that says *do no harm*, Morris says, "Cody very clearly taught me that harm for her would have been taking away that control. It would have been moving a hospital bed into her apartment. It would have been saying: You have to wait and linger in a state of unconsciousness or pain. And you have to know that your children and your family are going to watch the suffering. And for her, that would have been harm. So, what she taught me was that harm is different for every single one of us."

I very much admire Dr. Morris for her self-awareness in this situation. She recognized that any resistance she had to writing an aid-in-dying prescription for Cody stemmed from her own personal sense of loss. And ultimately, she was able to accept Cody's imminent death, work through her own grief and honor this request for the sake of her patient.

Supporting the Wishes of a Dying Loved One

In Chapter 3, I shared examples of how and why doctors and families surrounding the dying person can unwittingly encourage gross overtreatment or create other roadblocks to peaceful dying. But with patience and open conversation, the roadblocks can almost always be overcome. In addition to the heartening story of Dr. Morris and her patient Cody above, I'll share a few more stories of people who were able to put aside their personal qualms to help support, with loving intention, the wishes of a dying person.

Constance was a wife and mother of two who had spent more than a decade battling brain tumors. No longer able to walk, she was losing her ability to speak when she decided not to continue to deteriorate.

Constance wanted to have an honest conversation with her children, who were in their mid-to-late teens, before availing herself of medical aid in dying. She did not want them to learn of her decision after the fact. She feared that they would feel deceived and she also didn't want her husband to bear the burden of secrecy. Constance arranged counseling sessions to help her address these matters with her son and daughter. Unfortunately, both left midway through the first session and refused to return.

Bringing Constance's children back to the table was a daunting task. It took ten straight days of family visits, tears and difficult silences. Ultimately, love prevailed, and the children were able to move from denial to anger to acceptance of their mother's plan.

For her own part, Constance was enormously grateful to be open about her intentions, and to have her son and daughter with her, of their own free will, when she died. After Constance's death, both children said that although it was the most difficult thing they had ever done, they were glad to be able to give their mother one last gift of their support.

In another case, the roles were reversed, with a young man whose mother opposed his desire to stop treatment. Dave was a 26-year-old graduate student with an especially virulent form of cancer. Further treatment was unlikely to extend his life, but very likely to extend his suffering. Dave wanted to make the most of the time he had left.

At the time, Dave said, "I don't know if I'm going to apply for medical aid in dying. I just want my mother to understand why I might. She thinks if I accept what's happening to me and I stop fighting, it means I don't love her."

Gradually, this grieving woman came to accept that Dave would not return to the hospital for any cancer treatments and that his hospice chart would be updated with a DNR order. Bridging this impasse brought a deep relief. Dave reported that his relationship with his mother was much more relaxed and they were enjoying the remaining time together. He was grateful to experience this closeness with his mom and finally felt ready to die although, in the end, he decided not to pursue a request for medical aid in dying.

Constance chose medical aid in dying; Dave did not. But their hopes and expectations were the same. Each hoped that their doctors would listen deeply to what they valued most and explain how various treatment options would impact those values and priorities. Then, each expected that their physicians would support the choices they made and encourage all those who love them to do the same.

When Religion Places Obstacles

Another obstacle to a good death is the one so often posed by conservative religious leaders. I have little understanding of why it served some early religions to adopt the view that life, in any form, is always good and desired by God, and that death, in any circumstance, is always bad and shunned by God. After all, both life and death are part of the cycles set in motion at creation.

Nevertheless, we live with the harsh dual construct that any effort to preserve life, even a life devoid of consciousness or consumed by suffering, serves God and any effort to invite death, even a death both timely and desired by its conscious being, offends God. I don't adhere to this construct. But it is hardwired into every facet of our society and certainly manifest in the imperatives of our medical-industrial complex.

Thus we have the hard crux of the matter. The law and medical ethics are on the side of those who believe that to suffer, even needlessly, serves God, and they offer their suffering to their Lord. They are free to, and perhaps even encouraged to, remain in agony until the bitter and arbitrary end. But those who believe God's gift of life includes agency over that life, and who would choose to shorten the dying process when only agony remains, are on their own and made to feel "unlawful." Why, in a pluralistic nation, should some people be entitled to live their religious beliefs and others be required to live and die according to beliefs they do not share?

Though advocacy for medical aid in dying among clergy members is still more the exception than the rule in most parts of the nation, it has been my privilege to know many spiritual leaders who actively support the practice. In the early years, before more widespread social acceptance, a few thoughtful ministers stood out for their courage and candor. One is the Reverend Patricia Ross, Emeritus Minister of the United Church of Christ in Portland, Oregon.

Reverend Ross was ordained in 1982 after graduating from San Francisco Theological Seminary, and she received her Doctor of Ministry from Chicago Theological Seminary in 2001. She has publicly supported medical aid in dying since 1994. She has counseled dying congregants and other individuals on the theological aspects of choosing to abbreviate their dying process.

Reverend Ross tells the story of one such congregant, a young woman named Dawn who was dying from a brain tumor. At the time of her diagnosis, Dawn belonged to a very conservative Christian church, one whose close-knit community had long felt like family to her. As Dawn's pain became excruciating and her quality of life was vastly diminished, she sought her minister's counsel on whether to avail herself of Oregon's medical aid-in-dying option.

The minister told her in no uncertain terms that if she chose this path, she would be condemned to hell for all eternity. Dawn reported that he ordered the members of his congregation to have nothing to do with her until she had firmly resolved to "die according to God's plan." He warned them that to continue in relationship with her while she contemplated this sinful act would put their souls in jeopardy, as well. As a result, this dying young woman's support network abruptly withdrew.

Dawn eventually sought out Reverend Ross. The reverend recalls, "I talked with her about a loving God who wants people to be able to live and to have some joy and to have a real life. And yes, suffering is a part of life, but it's not a requirement that we suffer interminably. We talked for quite a long time about various passages in the Bible because Dawn was a very biblically literate person. In particular, we discussed Ecclesiastes, Chapter 3, Verse 2: *There is a time to be born and a time to die.*"

Dawn confessed that she and her boyfriend had hatched a desperate plan: Since he didn't believe in hell, he had agreed to push her off a bridge if it came to that. The idea was that he would be untroubled by any fear of eternal hellfire, and she would be innocent of suicide, since technically she would not have ended her own life.

"I don't know if Dawn had thought about what that would do to him!" Ross said. "If he loved her enough, I guess he was willing to do that. And that kind of determination and that kind of focus just shows how much this law is needed—that a person would go to that length to end his or her life."

Regarding the original pastor's stance, Ross reflected, "There is a belief among many Christians that there is something cleansing or strengthening or ennobling about suffering, or what I call redemptive suffering. There are times when people have suffered through some horrendous things and really gained some insight. But when you are talking about end-of-life suffering, in my mind, there comes a point when the suffering blots out any learning, insight or growth that might happen.

"Jesus said wonderful things about life and the meaning of life: *I come that you might have life and have it abundantly.* And when you get to the point where you cannot do anything, and you are in constant pain, when your body is just not responding to you in any way, that is not abundant life anymore."

Another religious leader who ardently supports medical aid in dying is Rabbi Ariel Stone of Congregation Shir Tikvah, also in Portland, Oregon. Rabbi Stone was ordained in 1991 by Hebrew Union College. In 2010, she completed her doctorate at the Spertus Institute of Jewish Studies. She served as President of the Oregon Board of Rabbis from 2007 to 2009. And in 2005, she testified to the Vermont State Legislature in support of a bill similar to Oregon's Death with Dignity Act.

"In my position, I have occasion to counsel both my own congregants and others who turn to me in their struggles with terminal illness," she told the Legislature. "As a rabbi, it is my duty to guide, but not to dictate, the final decision made by those whom I counsel. If someone chooses to exercise her right under Oregon's medical aid-in-dying law and she qualifies to use it, I have offered—and will continue to offer—my full support of that decision and help as I am able in the realization of that choice. This is my sense of the ethical imperative of my religious tradition."

Later in her testimony, she explained how, in her view, her stance conformed fully to her understanding of *halacha*, or Jewish law. "Oregon's Death with Dignity law reassures those who are nearing death that they need not be afraid, that death can be as good and as meaningful as life," she said. "This is a profoundly beautiful expression of the Jewish law that the dying are to be considered, for legal purposes, *khai l'kol davar*, 'like one who is alive for every purpose.' Not less than human, with their choices taken away and their dignity shredded, but worthy of the same respect and capable of wielding the same power over their lives until their very last moments as they did in their days of health, as all of us should have the right to do at every juncture of our lives. This, I submit, is what it truly means to "choose life" and to demonstrate the value of life, all the way through human life and to its end."

Forging Your Own Path

I deeply appreciate the ways in which many spiritual teachers understand their respective sacred texts as supportive of medical aid in dying. But perhaps my favorite perspective from a very devoutly religious figure comes from Dr. David Muller, an Orthodox Jewish doctor in the Compassion & Choices network of dedicated patient advocates. Not long ago I asked him, "When it comes to your patients' end-of-life decisions, what perspective do you bring as an Orthodox Jew?"

His answer was brief and blunt. "None," he said.

In response to my startled laughter, he added, "I hope that doesn't sound facetious. I don't mean it that way. But in my mind, in my role as a doctor, my own background plays no part whatsoever. It would be horrible, in my opinion, just terribly wrong for me to impose my own religious beliefs on a patient. It's the most absurd thing I can imagine. It isn't my job to make my patients comply with whatever course of action would feel right to me; it's my job to help them figure out and follow the path that feels right to them."

The issue really could be as blessedly simple as Dr. Muller has put it. The United States is not a theocracy. The first amendment in the U.S. Constitution declares that Americans may worship in any way they wish, or not at all. Physicians should not try to subvert that American value in their professional lives by forcing patients to conform to their personal religious beliefs. If they cannot accommodate a patient's freely chosen and legal choices, they should be swift to divulge that, and then should send their patients off with good wishes to a physician with a more tolerant moral philosophy.

Lessons from the Brittany Maynard Story

This ongoing debate between the tolerant and the dogmatic has never taken place on a more prominent stage than in the story of Brittany Maynard, who died from cancer in 2014, at the age of 30. Her death drew more awareness to the issues than any other event in the history of the movement for end-of-life options.

Brittany had a remarkable story and her telling of it changed everything for the movement. I recently told a reporter that I feel as though the decades that I had worked on these issues—from helping to draft and campaign for Oregon's Death with Dignity Act and putting it on the ballot in 1994 up until Brittany's story—had all been preparation for her emergence. That was the seminal moment. Brittany Maynard was the force that created enormous momentum within a brief time. At Compassion & Choices, she is hailed as a heroine.

Brittany was a beautiful, accomplished and breathtakingly vital woman. By her late twenties, she'd graduated from the University of California with a bachelor's degree in psychology and a master's degree in education. Spurred by a longtime interest in international travel, she taught at orphanages in Kathmandu, Nepal and traveled to Vietnam, Cambodia and other countries in Southeast Asia. She was happily married and enjoyed close relationships with her mother, her stepfather and many friends. She and her husband were about to begin their own family. But by late 2013, intense and frequent headaches had driven her to seek a medical evaluation that, by the first day of the following year, brought shattering news.

Her diagnosis was a grade 2 astrocytoma, a form of brain cancer. She was devastated to learn that her lifespan was likely to be as little as three years, but no more than ten. "I have to tell you, when you're 29 years old, being told you have that kind of timeline still feels like you're being told you're going to die tomorrow," she said.

She underwent a craniotomy and a partial resection of her temporal lobe, hoping to eradicate the tumor. But 70 days after surgery, an MRI dealt an even more dizzying blow. "I was told I had a grade change," she recalled. "[The doctors said] it looks like grade four, which is the worst and most aggressive form of brain cancer. It's called glioblastoma. So, that was a major shock to my system, and the system of my family, because I went from having potentially years of time to being told I had like six months."

Brittany's mother, Debbie Zeigler, offered a heart-wrenching description of the family's initial reaction. "In the beginning I hoped for everything," she said. "First, I hoped that they had just the wrong X-rays, the wrong set of scans, it was all just a big clerical mishap. Your brain will do really strange things to you when you don't want to believe something. You will come up with fairy tales."

And this is precisely what made Brittany so remarkable: her refusal to cling to this kind of denial or delusion, her grit and grace and clear-eyed sense of clarity. When the doctors prescribed full brain radiation in response to this new development, she researched both the side effects of this treatment and its likelihood to yield anything of value.

"The hair on my scalp would have been singed off," she said. "My scalp would be left covered with first-degree burns. My quality of life, as I knew it would be gone ... [Eventually] my family and I reached a heartbreaking conclusion: There is no treatment that would save my life, and the recommended treatments would have destroyed the time I had left."

Brittany's resolve to inform herself did not end there. She had the courage and the presence of mind to ask her doctors what her death would look like: what kind of symptoms she would have, what her experience would be like and what her family would have to witness. And the answers the doctors gave her only deepened her distress.

She was told that her seizures would become more frequent and longer in duration. She learned her headaches would intensify as the tumor swelled her brain and essentially crushed it against her skull, and that she would experience severe nausea and vomiting. She was likely to suffer strokes which would leave her with less and less bodily function. In their turn, she would lose her senses of smell, hearing and sight, and she'd lose the ability to move, followed by the loss of consciousness, until she finally died.

Brittany considered staying in hospice care at her San Francisco Bay–area home. But she knew that even with the best palliative care, she could develop morphine-resistant pain, experience personality changes and suffer physical and cognitive impairments of all kinds.

So, Brittany decided not to sign on for the grotesque and gratuitous suffering the tumor had in store for her. She thought: *It's enough that this cancer is taking me in the prime of my life, in the flower of my youth. I will not allow it to subject me—and my family—to horrific torture in the process.*

She researched her possibilities and made the decision to move to Oregon to avail herself of Oregon's authorization of medical aid in dying. She was thankful to have the resources and means to do this. Her husband was able to take a leave of absence from his work. Her mother was able to drop everything and accompany her on this move. And so, she, her husband, her mother and her step-father all moved to Oregon in June of 2014. Friends and extended family visited for long periods.

She proceeded to establish residency. She registered to vote. She obtained an Oregon driver's license. She found the best cancer care center in the state and established a relationship with physicians there so that she could continue the treatment options that seemed reasonable to her. She continued to search for new treatments and evaluate their success rate. She decided she wanted no aggressive measures with a low likelihood of prolonging her life and a high burden of side effects.

Meanwhile, she followed the procedures to qualify for aid in dying under the law. This is a considerable process, requiring repeated requests to two doctors, notification of options, mental capacity assessments, several waiting periods and completed and witnessed documents. Only after meeting numerous safeguards and overcoming barriers can a patient obtain an aid-in-dying prescription.

Brittany's physicians agreed she qualified. She was terminally ill, she had no more than six months to live, she was mentally competent and clearly under no duress from others. She was not suffering from clinical depression, nor was her judgment impaired in any way. She had been advised of all her alternatives. She'd considered and accepted other forms of comfort care. Once that evaluation was complete, the clock began on the fifteen-day period in which a second doctor had to independently assess her and draw all the same conclusions.

After two separate physicians had affirmed her eligibility, she had to fill out a formal request attesting to the same eligibility criteria and it had to be signed by witnesses. Then there was a mandatory second waiting period of 48 hours before a physician could finally write her a prescription for medication that would allow her to die peacefully in her sleep if she took it.

When Brittany became the most famous spokesperson of the end-of-life choices movement, it wasn't because she thought it her place to advocate for any one kind of death over another. It was because she passionately believed a dying person should be able to decide what kind of death would be the most fitting for his or her life story.

"I would not tell anyone else that he or she should choose death with dignity," she said. "My question is: Who has the right to tell me that I don't deserve this choice? That I deserve to suffer for weeks or months in tremendous amounts of physical and emotional pain?"

Unfortunately, this was not a rhetorical question and a predictable entity stepped up to assert its right to judge. Brittany took her medication and died peacefully, in her husband's arms November 1, 2014, two weeks before her 30th birthday. In the immediate wake of her death, the Vatican rendered its censure. Monsignor Ignacio Carrasco de Paula, head of the Pontifical Academy for Life, called Brittany's choice "reprehensible" and her means of death "an absurdity."

It took some time for me to take in the full force of this rigid and bitter condemnation. I had to sit for a time with the word *reprehensible*. As Brittany's family noted afterward, it's a very harsh word, unequivocal in its condemnation. This is the sort of word one might use to describe Nazi atrocities, crimes against humanity or the rape and abuse of children.

Terrorist acts, rape, murder, torture and slavery, human trafficking, brutality and genocide were raging around the globe. Amidst all this, the Vatican chose to focus its censure on a young woman who merely sought to make her imminent death a gentle one.

I wondered what, exactly, about Brittany's story the Monsignor judged as reprehensible. The resolve to stave off the most agonizing and pointless extremes of suffering that lay in store for her? The desire to spare her family the trauma of witnessing it? The choice to advocate for the many people at the same crossroads? Or was it, as I suspect, that she spoke in a prophetic voice of suffering and injustice, as all prophets do. She called attention to one of the ways government authority enforces what is essentially religious doctrine and tramples over our individual agency.

I would reserve the word "reprehensible" for those who intentionally harm others, perhaps even those who would heedlessly wound a grieving family in the immediate wake of their loss.

Meanwhile, which word in our lexicon would most precisely define the opposite of reprehensible? Whatever it is, Brittany's image is beside it in our dictionary. At Compassion & Choices, we are ever mindful of our gratitude to her. We speak of her with affection, we cherish her memory and we carry forth the torch she set ablaze.

Medical Interventions You Can Decline or Stop in Order to Die Peacefully, With Medical Support

- Renal dialysis
- Implanted defibrillator
- Ventilator, Bi-Pap or other breathing apparatus
- Cardiac pacemaker, for those with complete heart block
- Hi-tech cardiac support, such as an aortic pump
- Artificial feeding of any kind, via nasal tube, tubes in the stomach or other method
- Antibiotics for any infection, especially pneumonia
- Insulin, to induce diabetic coma
- Medication for congestive heart failure, but only with excellent comfort care to treat symptoms

Note: Death is not certain in every situation and deciding to stop any of these should be done only in close cooperation with your physician. Stopping any of these can lead to symptoms that may be distressing without supportive medical treatment.

11

Space for the Sacred

In 1996, I moved into the position of executive director of Compassion in Dying, a predecessor organization to Compassion & Choices. This position expanded my role in the end-of-life-choices movement, from that of an advocate to include service, as well. We were a staff of two and a volunteer crew of 11. For several years, until we grew large enough to add professional consultation staff, I talked with most out-of-state callers myself. Often, over the course of weeks or months, I gathered their stories, outlined their options and supported them in the choices they made. These were precious, intimate conversations, where people in the last phase of life eagerly shared their greatest fears, their deepest hopes and their path to acceptance and release.

Over and over, these individuals affirmed that dying is a psycho-spiritual experience as much or more than it is a physical one. This is especially true, I learned, for those who enter the process with a conscious presence and a desire for self-determination and intention. With my Unitarian Universalist outlook, it did not surprise me that devout religious belief and staunch personal autonomy could reside side-by-side in one psyche. But I did come to a greater appreciation that a sacred presence, however an individual conceives it, is often central and necessary for the healing and comfort of both the person dying and those facing imminent loss.

Those considering whether they wish to advance the time of death should not feel they must leave their religious tradition or spiritual beliefs behind. Instead, this is a time to revel in transcendent experience, call in our own angels of healing and compassion, stand in wonder at the great mystery and yield to the incomprehensible loving presence we have called "God." We should not feel shy or inhibited from inviting visitation from the divine or seeking luminous experiences. Sacred ritual, dreams, meditation practices, prayer, breathing techniques, music and song and even mind-altering substances can be invaluable in crafting life's closing chapter that is rich in traditional and personal spirituality.

In the late 1990s, Compassion in Dying was contacted by a family—Mary and her husband, Rodney, and their three adult daughters—looking for information and support.

Four years earlier, at the age of 74, Mary had noticed some subtle changes: loss of fine motor dexterity and poor balance. The family noticed slurred speech and thought perhaps some wine at dinner might be too much for someone her age. For months, Mary kept her fears of a brain tumor to herself. But when she began to stumble, and her handwriting deteriorated to scribbles, it was time to reveal her fears and visit a large research center for testing.

Tests revealed no tumor but also no other clear cause of her symptoms. For two years there was no diagnosis. But when she began falling over backwards without warning, losing peripheral vision and experiencing great difficulty speaking and writing, a neurodegenerative disease called progressive supranuclear palsy (PSP) was finally diagnosed.

PSP has no treatment, no cure, and the possibility of causing dementia in its final stages. Perhaps the most dismal part of Mary's diagnosis was that her intellect would stay fully intact through most of the physical deterioration. She just would not be able to speak or write or communicate.

By the late 1990s, PSP had rendered Mary mostly paralyzed, with rigid and contracted muscles, including those of the face. She was unable to stand, walk or speak clearly. The terminal phase of illness was at hand. After months of prayerful discernment and contemplation, Mary decided that the disease's final deterioration was worse than death and she wanted to end her life.

We at Compassion had the privilege to walk with this family through despair and grief, aided by their abiding religious faith and love for each other, to their noble and courageous actions. Almost twenty years later, this family still inspires me and exemplifies how approaching death with loving intention can become part of the family's story of love and religious commitment through adversity. Rodney and Mary's daughters, Jerri Lea, Merri Lea and Karen Lea, and the extended family have kindly allowed me to repeat some of their words and tell their story.

A Decision Made Lovingly, Thoughtfully, Prayerfully

Rodney and Mary grew up in Arkansas. As a teen during the depression, Rodney was so poor he stuffed newspaper in his shoes to cover the holes. His dad took on additional work and his mom took in boarders so they could send Rodney to college. Rodney earned money, too, by organizing and coaching a boxing team. To everyone's surprise, he and his team became so good they advanced to the quarterfinals in the national Golden Gloves tournament.

Mary grew up in the Southern Baptist Church and she, too, was able to attend college. That's where they met, though Rodney was two years ahead. He asked her out repeatedly before she said "Yes," and their dates consisted of his visiting her at her aunt's house, where she lived, and taking walks, chaperoned by Mary's young cousin on his bicycle. After dating six months, Rodney worked up the courage to kiss her. Madly in love after that, they never turned back.

Rodney and Mary adored each other, that was clear to everyone. Rodney celebrated their wedding anniversary every month on the 24th. The girls grew up hearing their dad announce at dinner how many months their parents had been married. (Years after Mary died, and Rodney's life was drawing to a close, his daughters told him they expected he would start counting when they met again.)

Rodney and Mary's life together was exhilarating, purposeful, infinitely loving and devoutly religious. It was as though their union did not merely add or multiply each other's energy, faith, altruism and buoyancy. Instead, their partnership expanded these qualities in the other exponentially. The list of causes they championed, organized and led is a long one. While still in college, Mary started a breakfast program for poor children. Together they integrated a college student YMCA/YWCA camp and started the first loan fund in the nation where students raised money and loaned it to anyone needing help to pay for college. They became leaders in the peace and social justice activities of every community they ever joined and readily started organizations to serve unmet needs as they discovered them. Their passion and commitment to building a better world were gifts they left to their daughters, and to us all.

For Mary, paralysis and confinement were torture, because service and activism were her spiritual practice and the meaning of her life. Her energy and activity were so much a part of her that decades before, when the family was moving east from Wisconsin, a group of Mary's friends wrote and performed a tribute play called *A Day in the Life of Mary* about her tirelessness. In the play, the day starts at 6:00 a.m. and ends at midnight, and along the way the character of Mary persuades more than a few people to vote and become involved in causes in the course of a day.

Throughout her life, Mary worked ceaselessly to promote women's participation in politics and enlist people in causes. So, inactivity felt like the death spiral it was, and this was a sacrilege to Mary. She yearned for escape.

Mary made her decision lovingly, thoughtfully, prayerfully. She would choose an earlier death over the imprisonment of her body and the relentless terminal deterioration. She asked her family if they would support her. Together they sought spiritual guidance through their minister, sacred texts and prayer. They called Compassion in Dying and we responded with empathic understanding, concrete information and emotional support.

Mary knew she would need a large quantity of sleeping medication, secobarbital, to carry out her plan. She would need to obtain it before her disease prevented her from swallowing it. This was a challenge, because Mary was growing weaker by the day.

I don't know exactly how she did it, but Mary eventually came into possession of the means to arrest her physical decline and time her death. Relief flooded over her and she relaxed into the circle of love surrounding her. She began to anticipate meeting her Lord in a place beyond this material world.

Mary's relationship with God, and her faith in God's love stands in stark contrast to common accusations that the movement for end-of-life choice is incompatible with spiritual practice or belief in divine presence. When journalists ask religious commentators why medical aid in dying happened first in Oregon, they often answer that fewer people in Oregon attend church than in any other state. This has always seemed like an attempt to disparage Oregonians and make them seem different from other Americans. "Those people are Godless and immoral" is the not-so-subtle message.

The overwhelming majority of Americans worship a supreme spiritual being, according to Gallup polls. Most call this power or being "God" and believe it shapes their lives in concrete ways. Oregonians are no different on this score. But those who oppose end-of-life choices are wrong in trying to equate regular church attendance with moral character. In 1998, one physician, a vocal opponent of medical aid in dying, told the *Dallas Morning News* that Oregon has "a greater moral deficit than the other states." Of course, his accusation of immorality is absurd, but so is the assumption that people who employ medical aid in dying have no religious faith or spiritual beliefs.

Religious Beliefs Are Intensely Individual

My experience is that Mary, and others like her, approach enormously difficult decisions with discernment and courage, and often with prayer. I have witnessed the task of preparing for death ennoble people of great integrity and draw loving families even closer together. Vibrant spiritual passion and deep religious beliefs often come to the fore.

One patient, whose church condemns assisted dying, expressed the certainty that her God would be waiting to greet her into heaven. Another, who knew her illness meant eventual suffocation, declared that, "God wouldn't want me to suffer like that." One husband, a Native American shaman, traveled to a sacred spot on Mount Shasta. As his wife took medication to hasten her death from breast cancer, he employed ancient rituals and prayers to ease her spirit across the borders of this life. As her family described it, he "drummed her spirit safely across to the other side."

In 2001, I spent a week at Ghost Ranch, in New Mexico, in dialogue with a community of religious scholars and devout, thoughtful individuals. During a discussion of this very issue one minister responded by saying, "Who knows the mind of God? Might not God also be working deliberately through those who *do* choose to end their lives?"

Religious beliefs are intensely individual, shaped by one's culture, background and personal experience of the divine. Everyone deserves to encounter death in a manner consistent with the values and beliefs they have come to cherish. "All religions must be tolerated," said Frederick the Great, "for every man must get to heaven his own way."

One church, the Catholic Church, leads the professional and political opposition to intentional dying—any act or omission with the intention to cause death. This includes both discontinuation of life-sustaining treatment, like feeding tubes, and voluntary ingestion of medication enabling a death during sleep. Because the National Conference of Catholic Bishops and its political conferences in each state are so vocal and visible in their opposition, people assume every religious denomination has the same attitude. This is not the case.

The firmness of Catholic doctrine on the issue of "intending" death is unique. I am no biblical scholar, but those who are scholars have taught me that no biblical text specifies or mandates such a doctrine. It was St. Augustine, in the fifth century, not Christ's

Apostles, who argued that the commandment "thou shalt not kill," applied to any act that hastened death. In the Middle Ages St. Thomas Aquinas reinforced this view and extended it to causing one's own death: "Whoever takes his own life sins against God ... for it belongs to God alone to pronounce sentence of death and life." It's important that some biblical scholars cite the Commandment in the original Aramaic as "Thou shalt not murder," which is not so broad as to render all intentional acts that end human life a violation of the Commandment.

Early Catholic theologians aside, the primary material of the bible is non-judgmental on the issue of intentional death. Reverend Madison Shockley, pastor of the Pilgrim United Church of Christ in Carlsbad, California, illustrates this with the story of King Saul, wounded and overtaken in battle against the Philistines. As the story goes, the Philistines were known for the torture and humiliation they inflicted upon prisoners captured on the battlefield. That is why, as they approached Saul, he commanded his armor bearer, "Draw your sword and thrust me through with it." Only through death could Saul avoid such suffering and degradation. The sword bearer refused, so Saul "took his own sword and fell upon it." The bible does not condemn Saul. In fact, it reports that after the Philistines desecrated Saul's body and fastened it to a wall, "all the valiant men" of Saul's kingdom set out and traveled all night to give him an honorable burial. They seized the bodies of Saul and his sons, burned them and buried the bones beneath a tamarisk tree.

Rev. Shockley goes on to draw an analogy between the Philistines and cancer, or other disease, that disintegrates the body and destroys its functions. Like Saul, a person might rationally choose death rather than undergo the humiliation, degradation and suffering their disease has in store for them in its natural course. If they do, the story of Saul seems to say that causing one's own death can be an act of honor. There is no sin here, in the eyes of God. Augustine and Aquinas are primarily responsible for the Catholic canons that death is evil and intending death is always immoral. A more compassionate theology regards death not as evil, but natural, and sometimes welcome in the face of extreme suffering.

William Herbert Carruth captures the universality of spiritual experience in this poem, written in 1902. It is remarkable for including Socrates' intentional death in its litany of the sacred.

Each in His Own Tongue

A fire-mist and a planet,

A crystal and a cell,

A jelly-fish and a saurian,

And caves where the cave-men dwell;

Then a sense of law and beauty

And a face turned from the clod—

Some call it Evolution,

And others call it God.

A haze on the far horizon,

The infinite, tender sky,

The ripe tint of the cornfields,

And the wild geese sailing high—

And all over upland and lowland

The charm of the goldenrod—

Some of us call it Autumn,

And others call it God.

Like tides on a crescent sea-beach,

When the moon is new and thin,

Into our hearts high yearning

Come welling and surging in—

Come from the mystic ocean.

Whose rim no foot has trod—

Some of us call it Longing,

And others call it God.

A picket frozen on duty,

A mother starved for her brood,

Socrates drinking the hemlock,

And Jesus on the rood;

And millions who, humble and nameless,

The straight, hard pathway plod—

Some call it Consecration,

And others call it God.

Most modern Christians affirm love, not life, as the ultimate Christian value. Death may come as a blessing to loving individuals in extreme circumstances. Devout thinkers of many faith traditions find little difficulty imagining actions that, taken carefully and prayerfully, might shorten life in the service of love.

Reverend Ralph Mero, one of the founders of Compassion in Dying, often described God's gift of life as, "more a loan than a gift." Nothing but temporary earthly life is ever received, and we have an absolute expectation that the loan will come due and the note will be called in. What lender is offended by early repayment, especially if the recipient has received the gift gratefully and used it well, for the good of all? A more generous and inclusive spirituality might also draw from ancient wisdom of the divine feminine, Native American, Hindu and other religious traditions less imbued with the good versus evil duality. Most ancient traditions and mythologies honor diverse aspects of divine power, including forces of creation, forces of protection as well as forces of destruction.

When we ask those who call upon Compassion & Choices, for help in dying, about their beliefs, most answer that they are either "religious" or "spiritual." Char Andrews, a client who helped us defend Oregon's law at the U.S. Supreme Court, told reporters, "I think it's more spiritual to die before I'm comatose, with my family and loved ones at my bedside." An Episcopal priest with stage-four cancer told us his religion greatly influenced his choice. He found no conflict between his faith and his desire to end his life if suffering became a needless cruelty. "I worship the God who is the lover of souls and hates God's and humanity's enemies—suffering and cruelty—and only wills the best for me."

Finding Support During Illness and Death

Rodney and Mary's church, their pastor and their faith sustained them through the ordeal of Mary's illness and death. Rodney was theologically trained himself, having served as an army chaplain in the European theater during World War II and later, having obtained a divinity degree from Garrett Biblical Institute in Illinois. For three years, he rode a circuit of rural churches in Wisconsin, preaching to five small congregations every Sunday. When Rodney tired of that, he received permission to leave the pulpit and work full-time for world peace. They were dedicated and prominent members of their church community, and through three official retirements, Rodney continued to be active in Dumbarton's Peacemakers/PeaceSeekers. They were especially close to their pastor, the Rev. Dr. Mary E. Kraus.

All this confirmation of religious devotion is not to say her illness did not test Mary's faith in a benevolent god. It did. As her disease took hold, Mary wondered why God would punish her with an illness that had no cure or treatment, that would take everything from her before claiming her life. Rev. Kraus saw her through this crisis with attentive pastoral care.

It was during this spiritual struggle that Rev. Kraus began visiting their home every Sunday afternoon. In these, "Sundays with Mary," Rev. Kraus supported Mary in an ancient and profound spiritual quest. Because Mary had trouble speaking, Rev. Kraus would often articulate questions and Mary would answer with squeezes of the hand. Rev. Kraus told others that, "Sheer grace led to the formation of each question as the two were discovering that God was indeed present in the midst of this turmoil and suffering."

For those looking for support similar to what Rev. Kraus provided to Mary, I suggest Rabbi Harold Kushner's best-selling book, *When Bad Things Happen to Good People*, which has similarly supported countless people through grief and offered healing through tragedy. In continuous print since its publication in 1981, the popularity of this book attests to our need to make sense of human suffering and transcend it.

A United Purpose

A second crisis of doubt visited the family in the days before Mary died. This time it was doubt of each other.

Mary stopped being anxious once she had collected the required amount of sleep medication. She instructed the family to put it in a safe place until she knew the time was right to ingest it. Rodney and the daughters were grateful Mary wasn't eager to take it immediately, so they were happy to put it out of sight. Thus began a period of review and celebration for Mary. She made a list of things she wanted to do to celebrate her life—return to places she adored, eat her favorite dishes brought from her favorite restaurants, wheel through the park with grandchildren running beside her and swim with her three daughters, one at a time, in her aquatic therapy sessions.

Days passed. Then weeks. Mary didn't ask about the medication. The family didn't mention it. Everyone started to sense a strain in their interactions, a tension in the air, but no one understood why it was happening. Finally, they decided to consult their minister, hoping that pastoral counseling would reveal the difficulty and help overcome it.

Reverend Kraus came to the family's home and asked to speak with Mary alone. After some time alone with Mary, she then asked to speak with Rodney and the daughters, out of Mary's hearing. Alone with their pastor, Mary and her family were separately able to express what weighed on their hearts.

Mary told her minister that she was ready to take her medication. She feared missing her window of opportunity, when she was still able to hold fluid in her mouth and swallow it. She wanted her family to give her permission to leave them. She hesitated to ask because she didn't want them to think she didn't love them enough to stay or that she didn't appreciate the love and attentiveness she received from them every day.

For their part, Rodney and the daughters also realized that soon Mary would be too weak to swallow, but they dared not mention this to her, for fear she might think they were urging her to take the medication. So, each remained silent for the others' sake, and misunderstanding grew.

Reverend Kraus brought the family together and explained each set of concerns. Each now understood how silence had entrapped them. The family was together again, in united purpose to give Mary what she wanted, to honor her wish to end her life with grace and comfort, and soon.

Sacred Rituals on the Chosen Day

The family made plans to gather the family on Mary's chosen day. They began to plan a sacred ritual for that day. They read to her a passage from a book called *The Bond Between Women, a Jour-*

ney to Fierce Compassion, by China Galland, because it reflected Mary's indomitable spirit, her faith and her dedication to the women of Central America.

> There is a goodness, a Wisdom that arises, sometimes gracefully,
>
> sometimes gently, sometimes awkwardly, sometimes fiercely,
>
> but it will arise to save us if we let it,
>
> and it arises from within us,
>
> like the force that drives green shoots to break the winter ground,
>
> it will arise and drive us into a great blossoming like a pear tree,
>
> into flowering, into fragrance, fruit and song,
>
> into the wild wind dancing, sun shimmering,
>
> into the aliveness of it all,
>
> into that part of ourselves that can never be defiled,
>
> defeated, or destroyed, but that comes back to life,
>
> time and time again, that lives—always—that does not die.
>
> Into the Divine.

Rodney, the daughters and their husbands were all there, of course. So was Reverend Kraus. Their simple and poignant ritual began with the gathering in a circle. They went around the circle, greeting each other with the words, "God's spirit rests upon you." Rev. Kraus offered a reading and each family member shared a brief word with Mary, telling her how she had blessed their lives and wishing her a safe journey. Rev. Kraus gave a blessing and a concluding prayer.

After this ceremony and tender goodbyes, Rodney was the last to lean in and kiss his wife farewell.

But he was playful to the end. Everyone knew one of Rodney's favorite jokes was about a woman who died and, soon after entering heaven, became responsible for tending the pearly gates. She had heard St. Peter ask people to spell "love" before allowing them in.

Well, who appeared at the gates but her husband. He exclaimed with delight when he saw her, ecstatic that they would spend eternity together.

"Not so fast," she said. "You have to spell a word."

"What word?" he asked eagerly.

"Czechoslovakia," she replied.

After kissing Mary, Rodney leaned in closer and whispered to his wife, "Now, remember, the word is LOVE, not Czechoslovakia."

With that settled, Mary drank the medication and quickly slipped into a deep sleep. Her face took on a liveliness they had not seen in years and a peaceful glow surrounded her.

Her loved ones kept vigil around the bed. One sang a familiar hymn, another cradled her body, another told a story. When her breathing stopped, they shared a comforting reading. Rodney stayed with Mary all night, leaving only after he felt certain her spirit had gathered itself completely and left her body.

Rodney: A Social Justice Warrior

When I finally met Rodney face to face we had already spoken by phone many times and corresponded by mail. We had planned my visit while his beloved Mary was still alive, but we anticipated her time was close. I wrote that I hoped to see him during my trip to Washington D.C. in early December, and acknowledged, "Your heart may be breaking at that time."

Indeed, when he and I embraced on meeting, I saw that though his heart was breaking, it was also filled with gratitude that his beloved had gotten her wish and suffered no more.

Rodney brought out the family photo albums. He wanted me to see his Mary through the years and know her story. There was the photo of Mary as a girl, standing with her big family outside the two-room house with the plank floor where she grew up. There were their wedding pictures and photos of their girls as each arrived, and photos of milestones passed as they grew up.

I learned more about Rodney's story on that day, too. I learned he was one of 22 whites on the 54-mile Selma march and that he still felt enormously honored to have taken every blistering step of witness. Afterwards, he organized clergy nationwide to rebut racist attacks on the march and even took on the mayor of Selma in a televised David Susskind debate.

Rodney called one exchange in the debate his "greatest comeback ever." The mayor asked Rodney if he didn't think ministers had "better get out of political and social revolution and get back to saving souls? Would Jesus advocate civil disobedience?" To which Rodney replied, without hesitation, "I don't think he was crucified for obeying the law."

On a different issue, Rodney had directed both his fury and his strategic mind toward a Congressman from West Virginia who blocked a bill to provide birth control to low-income women. Rodney organized Methodist women in that Congressman's district. With his encouragement, they never let up until that bill became law.

I felt honored and grateful when Rodney added the campaign to authorize medical aid in dying to his list of social justice concerns. With characteristic energy and good humor, he set about bringing people to our cause, as he had so many others. He scheduled talks in churches and homes, wrote letters and opinion pieces and told Mary's story over and over.

It was fun and exciting to join Rodney in a presentation, as he made people laugh and cry and almost always won them over. And he never failed to ask attendees to support our work with a financial contribution. He knew money was the necessary fuel for any successful movement and he wasn't shy about asking for it.

Shaping a Spiritual Narrative at the End of Life

One advantage of an intended death is that it doesn't take people by surprise. The individual who is dying has time to perform the tasks of life completion. Families have time to travel and attend to the one whom they will soon lose. Everyone can access and benefit, together or individually, from the transformative power of ritual and the healing power of community and family ties. A life coming to closure can provide a profound and sacred lesson in how to live.

Here is the opportunity to shape not only a heroic narrative, but also a spiritual narrative, at the end of life. Shared memories, healing words, poems, prayers, music and laughter can create a spiritual experience that, like any sacred ritual, changes people. There's a ripple effect when a holy event is planned and witnessed. The love and grace experienced in the moment get carried into the world as part of the life story of everyone present. Sacred ritual does not merely mark an event, it changes those who participate in that event.

In 1995, Rabbi Zalman Schachter-Shalomi published *From Ageing to Sage-ing: A Revolutionary Approach to Growing Older,* a book designed to help people prepare for advancing age, extreme old age and death with more anticipation than dread, more gratitude than grief. I think of this work as sacred work, work we were born to do, work that, when neglected, will keep us from achieving the joy in life and the sense of completion at death that are our birthright.

Zalman already had a lifetime of innovation behind him, being one of the founders of the Jewish Renewal movement and an innovator in ecumenical dialogue. His book laid the foundation for a movement variously called "sageing," "conscious aging" or "conscious eldering." He remained its revered leader until his death in 2014 at the age of 89. Rabbi Zalman starts with the premise that mortality is our teacher in being more generous, loving and joyful as we age. "Death," he writes, "is *not* a cosmic mistake. Woven into the warp and woof of existence, the presence of death deepens our appreciation of life. It also regenerates our psyches in preparation for harvesting." The conscious aging movement could be called a life-affirming movement in death preparation, for that, at its core, is what it is.

Ideally, we would all follow Zalman's advice and undertake the tasks of life completion long before our own ending comes into view. Certainly, it's never too late to start, and we will find the enterprise surprisingly enlivening. Even if we delay, much of what he teaches can help make our last weeks or months of life a time of vastly expanded consciousness. Many terminally ill people do report finding a measure of joy, serenity and gratitude that remains remarkably elusive until we come to number our days in a concrete way.

In 2000, Bill Moyers produced a stunning documentary series on death called *On Our Own Terms*. During one episode, he followed a terminally ill physician who spoke of his appreciation for the glorious beauty of spring, when he had not expected to see another. Never do I behold April's exhilarating explosion of azaleas, rhododendron and dogwood that I don't hear this man's words in my ear. I hear his words as a pressing reminder of a more benevolent version of the shrouded specter of death, who commands from gravestones, "Live . . . for I am coming."

Rabbi Zalman and others explain the tasks of life completion and describe exercises and meditations to accomplish them. The first task, and one that often comes naturally, is life review. Looking at old photographs and telling stories is not merely idle memory. As we do these things we also harvest the fruits of a lifetime of experience and relationship. Not all these fruits are tasty, of course, and we will no doubt find some quite bitter. But each carries a bit of the history of our heart, the "soul's code," in the words of psychologist James Hillman.

It's amazing how often patterns and insights emerge in a life review to reveal a deeper meaning and purpose. Through this exercise we come to appreciate the shape of our individuality. Here we may discover, or recognize for the first time, the "call" in our life, or the fate that placed it in some greater context of history and human behavior. As we view life in retrospect, our errors and omissions magically turn into lessons and insights, often to our delight. Spanish poet Antonio Machado captures a wonderful image in his poem, "Last Night As I Was Sleeping." The poet dreams a "marvelous error," a "beehive, here inside my heart," where, "the golden bees were making white combs and sweet honey from my old failures."

Forgiving Yourself and Others at the End

Forgiveness is another important task. This entails forgiveness of ourselves for the multitude of past errors, and forgiveness of others who have harmed us.

Human frailty being universal, no one gets through life without accumulating a mountain of transgressions, errors, oversights, acts of greed, neglect or ignorance. Many of us indulge in mental drumbeats of internal criticism, beating ourselves up endlessly for all these shortcomings. Old age and terminal illness are the time to finally give all that up, if somehow we have not already yielded to a kinder tolerance. As poet Mary Oliver writes, "When will you have a little pity for every soft thing that walks through the world, yourself included?"

Sallirae Henderson writes of the importance of "befriending yourself" in her brilliant book, *A Life Complete*. To befriend yourself, she explains, is to treat yourself as you would expect a friend to treat you. A friend tolerates imperfection. A friend may offer helpful observations but does not berate you needlessly. A friend reinforces your essential decency and loves you for your imperfections.

Forgiving others may be the more vital task. "Forgiveness work," Rabbi Zalman writes, "challenges us with the evolutionary task of ennobling our sufferings, transmuting tragedy and sorrow to understanding and the capacity to love." The stakes are high if we fail to forgive, for the alternative to forgiveness is confinement in a cramped and bitter prison of resentment, where no one would wish to die.

Truly, some things are unforgivable in their cruelty or depravity. So, we must understand that to forgive does not mean to pardon or condone. It does mean to reconcile and come to a place of reconciliation for our own sake, not for the sake of the one who wronged us. The work is "for" my own "giveness." The question is, "Can I get to the point where I can be a 'giving person' again, in spite of the terrible injustice, pain or loss I have suffered?" Remorse from the one who hurt us is often key to reaching a state of reconciliation.

Two inspiring examples are South Africa's Truth and Reconciliation Commission and Rwanda's recovery from the horrific genocide of its minority Tutsi population. Tutsi survivors say of the Hutu neighbors, "When they asked to be forgiven, we could, because we could see it was coming from their hearts." Today Hutu and Tutsi people live side by side again in harmony and work together to manifest the motto of post-genocide reconciliation, "Never again."

Rodney and His Intentional Death

In his 89th year, Rodney, Mary's widower, had no unfinished business. The stories and patterns of his life had become a well-worn cloth, familiar as an old sweater, comforting as a warm shawl. He had lived his faith in tireless work for peace and justice over seven decades. He had long since transferred a keen social consciousness on to his children. He had taught them well. In their house "love your neighbor," and "help the less fortunate," were said as often as "brush your teeth," or "finish your homework."

Anger or resentment had never found a resting place in Rodney's heart, and forgiveness and reconciliation were an established habit. He had stretched the limits of activism when he rode a wheelchair through an entire march for women's lives two years before. He had already tithed most of his assets to organizations working for peace, disarmament and population control. But now, after nine decades, Rodney was getting weaker, losing the ability to do the things that gave him purpose and joy. He was ready to die.

Once again, Reverend Mary Kraus gave pastoral counsel and Rodney felt firm in his faith and right with his god. Rodney and I talked about how he might accomplish a peaceful death and he settled on a plan. For several years, Rodney had lived with a defibrillator implanted in his heart, because he was prone to a lethally abnormal heart rhythm. Periodically, damaged cells in his heart discharged erratic electrical impulses that disrupted the normal pacing function. Left alone, his heartbeat would deteriorate into the shuddering motions of ventricular fibrillation, totally ineffective to pump blood to vital organs. The implanted device sensed this happening before Rodney would otherwise lose consciousness, and it delivered an electric shock that restored the heart's normal rhythm and function.

Rodney hated when this happened. The abnormal rhythm itself was painless, but the shock was excruciating. He lived in constant fear of the abrupt agony caused by the firing of this internal device. Rodney decided to have the cardiologist deactivate the implanted defibrillator. Then, the next time his heart went into ventricular tachycardia and fibrillation, he would die, swiftly and painlessly.

In 2015, about 160,000 Americans had defibrillators implanted, more than double the number from the prior decade. Instead of dying suddenly from the heart's fibrillation, now patients with an internal defibrillator are much more likely to die slowly in a struggle for breath as congestive heart failure fills their lungs with fluid. Still, few patients deactivate the devices, and cardiologists don't like to turn their machines off. But Rodney insisted. He argued that the pain and suffering from being subjected to electric shocks was too great a burden to bear. The pain outweighed the meager benefit of prolonging a life that was severely compromised and nearing its natural end.

Rodney arranged for the decommissioning of his life-prolonging device. Once again, the family prepared to journey together through the bright sadness of losing one of their beloved. They gathered in abundant love and generous spirit and agreed to

Rodney's plan.

On the day Rodney chose for what he called his "Great Amen," Reverend Kraus, family and friends gathered in a ceremony to honor him, bless him and invoke the spirit of boundless love to accompany him. Like the ceremony for Mary, it included the elements that bring participants into a time and place that feels holy. It invoked eternal, universal themes of transcendence and mystery. It used poetry and music to tap into the human response to rhythm, art and language. It named that for which we are grateful and called them "blessings." And it ended with a parting wish for understanding, loving kindness or peace that we call "prayer."

As Kathy Black explains in her book of ritual resources for women called *Wising Up,* this type of ritual at the very end of life should follow much conversation and prayerful consideration between participants and pastor. Everyone should feel nourished by a sacred ritual and if anyone is not comfortable with it, they should not feel forced to participate. Every ceremony should be tailored to the needs and desires of the people involved.

Black offers these questions as an example of what a pastor or other officiant might ask the individual for whom it is intended and their family:

- **What** do you want or need to say at this time to your spouse/mother/friend? Are there stories that haven't been shared or words of love and thanks and goodbye that still need to be said or need to be said one last time?
- **What** readings (scripture, quotations, poetry) would be comforting in the person's last hour?
- **What** music or songs might evoke memories and pleasure?
- **What** prayer language might dwell within so that peace may abide, and God's presence be felt during the journey of crossing over?
- **How** should the various elements be ordered?
- **How** will the group gather? Informally or with some

formal greeting?

- **What** opening words will be used? An opening prayer, a song or reading of some sort? Or will the family begin immediately with sharing their stories and saying their words of love, thanks and goodbye?
- **What** symbols will be present? Candles, incense, photos, a favorite quilt, a stuffed animal from a grandchild? What will the room look like? What meaningful elements of the [person's] life will be visually present for this moment?
- **Who** will give the blessing (if any)? From family members to the [dying person] and/or (if the [dying person] is capable) from him or her to the family members?
- **How** will the ritual end? With a prayer? A benediction?
- **Passing** of the Peace to the [dying person] and to each other?

Rituals can be very simple. The 2011 documentary film *How to Die in Oregon* followed Cody Curtis (previously mentioned on page 198) and her family through the last days of her decline from liver cancer and her ultimate death, enabled by Oregon's medical aid-in-dying law. Hers was a musical family and their natural inclination was to express spiritual themes in song. Cody drank her medication in her own bed, with her family attending her.

As she drifted to sleep, the last sounds she heard were of those who loved her, singing the classic hymn "I'll Fly Away."

Some glad morning when this life is o'er,

I'll fly away.

To a home on God's celestial shore,

I'll fly away.

I'll fly away, oh glory, I'll fly away.

When I die, Hallelujah, by and by,

I'll fly away...

Celebrating Rodney's "Great Amen!"

Rituals for passing are as different as the individuals for whom they are prepared. Families and clergy alike may find it helpful to have an example of a ceremony like this in full, one that was prepared for an intentional death. Reverend Mary Kraus and the family constructed a powerful and poignant ritual that is an excellent example. Below, I include the outline and script for Rodney's "Great Amen" ceremony. The words were spoken by Rev. Kraus, who officiated.

Celebrating Rodney's "Great Amen!" • January 27, 2006

Gathering the Circle

This is Rodney's special day. It is a day that has taken a lifetime of living and it has now arrived. We gather as family to share this together and to journey with you, Rodney, as far as our lives permit.

(To Rodney)

I think Paul's words help articulate the understanding of life that you have so wonderfully shared with all the rest of us.

If we live, we live for the Lord; and if we die, we die for the Lord.

Whether therefore we live or die, we belong to the Lord. (Romans 14:8)

(To the Family)

One of the things this family does so well is storytelling. Now because of the way Rodney and Mary lived their lives, you have created a lot of stories—few of which are dull! The other thing is that Rodney keeps teaching us that life is full of humor. It may not always be easy, but if one is truly living, there will always be laughter.

Now, Rodney, there will be some tears here because we know we are going to miss you. So, as we share some of our favorite stories, we will all laugh but we may also be passing the Kleenex box now and then—that is just to give a little warning of our behavior and I am sure you will remind us if we seem to be losing touch with humor. So, I invite each of us now to share a "Rodney" story, if you are so moved.

Sharing of Favorite Stories—all participate

These are but a taste of the stories your lives have written in relationship to Rodney as father, father-in-law, grandfather, uncle, friend. And Rodney, when your heart stops beating, you will live on in many ways and one of them will be through the stories. Once again, our brother Paul who lived so long ago speaks to us:

There is nothing in death or life, in the world as it is, or the world as it

Shall be, nothing in all creation, that can separate us from the love of

God in Christ Jesus our Lord. (Romans 8:38-39)

Giving Rodney a Blessing

As we told these stories, it is clear that you have been a blessing to not only us, but to many, many others. And we want to offer you some blessings now, as we send you on your way. (One person offered the blessing of Rodney's work continuing after him. Another blessed him in his remarkable ability to spell whatever word Mary or anyone else ever asked him to spell. Another blessed him with the reminder that just as he has been teaching us that life and death are inseparable—and one can be joyously ready for death—that blessing now returns to him as he completes his earthly journey.)

Anointing Rodney for His Journey

Rodney, I anoint your head with this oil of forgiveness, healing and salvation. You have thought many thoughts, some of which were spoken! You have dreamed dreams and seen visions, some of which irritated lots of folks and some of which empowered justice to be seen in our midst.

I anoint your hands and feet which have taken you many miles, stuffed many envelopes, shaken many hands, written many speeches, run the good race and held the life-line for people with no hope.

I anoint your heart which has sustained your life for 88 years, loved Mary and your three daughters, and later your growing circle of family. It is from your heart that you wrote and spoke of God's love for all people, not just for some. It is from your heart that you addressed the moral issues of each day. And it is your heart that now says it is tired and wants to rest.

God our Creator and our end, thank you for both life and death, and for your spirit of curiosity and adventurousness that dwells within Rodney. Give us the trust and confidence that he has, to know that it is into your peace he journeys. Amen.

I'd like to close with a poem for Rodney's "Great Amen!" Its words are to all of us—to Rodney at the close of this earthly journey and to us as we continue until the day arrives when we also complete ours.

"Amen"

Be careful of simple words said often.

"Amen" makes demands like an unrelenting schoolmaster: fierce attention to all that is said, no apathy, no preoccupation, no prejudice permitted.

"Amen": We are present. We are open,
        We harken. We understand,
        Here we are; we are listening to your word.
"Amen": makes demands like a signature on a dotted line:
        Sober bond to all that goes before;
        No hesitation, no half-heartedness, no mental
        reservation allowed.
"Amen": We support. We approve.
        We are of one mind. We promise.
        May this come to pass. So be it.

Be careful when you say "Amen."

—*Barbara Schmich*
A Liturgy Sourcebook

Concluding Prayer

God of love, we thank you for that which you have blessed us with even to this day: for the gift of joy in days of health and strength, and for the gifts of your abiding presence and promise in the days of pain and grief. We praise you for each person in this family circle, and for all the friends who have expanded the circle over the years. We offer special thanks for Rodney who has made sure that his daughters grew up knowing that they were strong and gifted individuals and that life was full of adventure and for his faithful presence to each one gathered here.

Amen! (said by everyone)

Opening of the Circle—Let Rodney Pass Through

We open our circle now so that Rodney may get ready to go to the doctor. It is your pilgrimage, Rodney, and we will go with you as far as we can. But this is really your journey. May you go well.

Rodney went directly from this ceremony to his cardiologist's office, where the doctor de-activated the implanted defibrillator. Rodney was expecting to die right then and there, but he did not die. In order for his plan to work, his heart had to go into its lethal rhythm, and instead, it kept beating away like clockwork.

So, Rodney went home, with hospice care, and resumed his life. Without the constant fear of being jolted by an electric shock, he was more relaxed. He continued to take regular meals, enjoy talking with family and friends, and express gratitude to his nurses. Nine days later, Rodney died naturally, fully expecting to see his beloved Mary again, and knowing exactly how to spell Czechoslovakia.

Elements of a Ritual of Celebration of a Life About to End

A formal officiant, like a minister or an informal one, like a family member, may serve as leader.

- **A sacred environment.** Arrange the space clear of distraction. Mark the beginning of the ritual with words, a chime or bell. Form a circle or have participants face the dying individual.

- **Invocation.** Set the intention, state the purpose of the ceremony.

- **Readings.** These may be scripture, poems, story or meaningful prose.

- **Story-telling.** Participants reminisce, tell stories that reflect the life that is coming to a close.

- **Music.** People may sing together, or just listen. Any kind of music is appropriate, and the choice will be highly individual.

- **Prayer, or statement of wishes and hopes.** These can be for the one who is dying and for those who will continue their earthly journey without this person's presence.

- **Saying goodbye.** Opportunity for each person to say a few words of farewell.

- **Concluding blessing.** This can also be a statement of comfort or acceptance of nature's cycles of life and death.

12

It's Harder Than
You Think
(But We Can Do It)

My professional life began in nursing. And though I left nursing for medicine, law and policy four decades ago, in a sense I've "been a nurse" since 1970. Being a nurse taught me about living and dying and informed every endeavor I've undertaken since.

Before nursing school, I had very little exposure to serious illness. But that changed early in my education. Cornell University-New York Hospital School of Nursing occupied a stately building on the east side of Manhattan, adjacent to the New York Hospital. People came from all over the world to be treated at this renowned institution and their relatives occasionally stayed in the nursing dorm.

One night, I was awakened by the keening of a woman using the phone in the hallway. Her grief was raw and immediate, and I remember the stricken ache that took root in my chest as I listened to her sobs. I sensed that I had chosen work which would bring me regularly to the sharp edges of human experience. I felt awed by that, and grateful for the privilege that came with it: an intimate familiarity with the depths of human experience.

In retrospect, nursing was the best possible apprenticeship for the balance of my life's work. Nursing kindled the torch of patient advocacy and today, as Compassion & Choices gathers unprecedented momentum, it burns as brightly as it ever has. Authorized aid in dying has brought immeasurable benefits to dying individuals—benefits like peace of mind, a sense of autonomy, the chance to die at home and an end to much needless suffering. Our organization has also done much to improve access to hospice and palliative care, ensure that patient wishes are heeded, and help patients avoid pointless and invasive procedures.

But in spite of these accomplishments, it seems we've barely begun. The need for medicine to change and the opportunity for it to change are both enormous. We now understand medical aid in dying as a catalyst that can set change in motion, to make medical encounters not merely patient-centered but *patient-directed*. Today, patients may be the center of attention and still have no authority or ability to assert their own values and priorities. Only when they get to **direct** their treatment will it align with what matters most to them as they age, or as illness progresses.

"Hard" Is Not Impossible

It may indeed be harder than you think to achieve a peaceful death. But "hard" is not impossible. If this book does nothing else, I hope it persuades readers that the right kind of preparation *works*. We *can* live according to our values, beliefs and priorities as illness advances. We can die calmly in our own beds and leave peaceful memories for our loved ones. Knowing the risks of inaction can help. Developing new expectations, attitudes and habits can transform our own experiences and the entire field of medicine, too.

Many stories cross my desk of people whose desperation mounted as life ebbed and only agony flowed on, until they finally took independent action. For me the saddest stories are those of men with guns. So often it's the virile and the manly—the ones whose lives were one long round of taking charge, making plans and doing tasks—who die the hardest deaths. They may die violently and often alone. These are men who pride themselves on being prepared for any eventuality. As one such man once told me, "You know me, Barbara. I'm an eagle scout. 'Be prepared' is my motto."

This book does not suggest preparation involving a gun. Nor does it reiterate the preparations that are usually advised, because they are insufficient. Advance directives, end-of-life conversations, Do Not Resuscitate (DNR) orders: these are generally not helpful as illness insidiously advances, symptoms escalate, and acute deterioration appears on the horizon.

Slowly advancing illness is the most common situation we all encounter and handling that well can prepare us and our families for decisions about life support that may come later. The stakes are high. The kind of preparation I'm talking about is far different from what is usually meant by an "end-of-life conversation." Preparation for slow decline means adjusting our attitudes and expectations of the healthcare system and turning the system to our own needs.

The good news is it can be done, and the habits we acquire will serve us as long as we live. The bad news is we must do it ourselves, for doctors and hospitals are unlikely to do so. To play off a famous Pogo phrase, "We have met, not the enemy, but the solution, and it is us."

When There Isn't a Full-Range of Options for Peaceful Dying

As I have learned, even people who pride themselves on being prepared cannot be truly prepared if they are forced to do their planning alone and in secret. Without professional consultation and discussion of a full range of options for peaceful dying, they may turn to crude, unreliable or violent means of self-help. They endure the torment of lonely uncertainty and their loved ones face impossible questions of what may constitute the most loving, faithful and honorable course for them.

Alex Fraser, a Washington, D.C., entrepreneur, is an example of someone who put a great deal of thought and energy into being prepared. In fact, you could say his preparedness bordered on an obsession.

"He had gallons of water in his basement in case the water main were ever compromised," recalls his daughter Alexa. "A classic Christmas gift from my dad—a favorite stocking stuffer—was this multi-purpose survival device. It had a little hammer you could use to break your window if your car were submerged in a lake, and a razor blade, and many other tools for various emergencies. It was a device for the truly prepared person." Alex had even moved to Australia during the Cuban Missile Crisis and to Arkansas during Y2K, as his way to be prepared for the worst.

Fraser blazed a colorful, energetic and vibrant path wherever he went. He survived the toughest of what "The Greatest Generation" endured. He fought in the European theater during World War II and became a prisoner of war in Germany during its waning days. The German army had begun massacring American soldiers who surrendered, so the soldiers in his platoon expected the worst. He clung to hope when he arrived at the factory that was to be his prison and his captors gave him a crudely-made spoon. He took courage from his theory that they wouldn't waste a spoon on a soldier marked for death, and he was right.

In his later years, Fraser lived with a condition known as "essential tremor," which increased the likelihood that he would develop Parkinson's. Toward the end of his ninth decade, it became clear that it was indeed turning into Parkinson's. With this debility came a marked decrease in Fraser's quality of life, and after a certain point, his daughter was well aware that he was looking for a way to hasten his own death.

"Even before his decline, my father had long made it clear to me and to anyone else who would listen that if something bad were to happen to him, he wanted action taken to protect him from a life that was unacceptable to him," says Alexa. "And with the onset of his Parkinson's, he continually pressed me for reassurance that if, say, he fell in his house and then suffered in a nursing home, I would ensure that he wouldn't languish in that condition.

"If he weren't able to take the necessary actions to hasten his death, he wanted me to take those actions on his behalf. And while I wanted nothing more than to support my father in facing the end of his life on his own terms, of course I worried that fulfilling this request would make me vulnerable to legal repercussions. I mean, he had this idea that I could just turn off his respirator in the hospital and not report it, which of course was just not realistic."

Alexa reported that even after her father's life became extraordinarily difficult, and in spite of his stated desires, the family still observed a series of deeply meaningful milestones together. They celebrated Alex's 90th birthday. Alexa's son graduated from 8th grade and played a lead role in the school play. These events served as a series of "Things To Look Forward To." But after the last of these, without another on the horizon, Alex felt ready to depart.

"One afternoon, he told me over the phone that he was in a lot of discomfort and was going to take pain pills," Alexa says. "Naturally I thought he meant a single dose of pain pills, but I wasn't able to reach him the next morning. There was a woman in his area, a friend of mine, who checked on him regularly and she wasn't able to reach him either. So, she went over there. She had a key to his house, but the chain was on the door. She was able to hear him, though. He called to her from inside to break the chain, and she did."

Alex was lying on the couch. He had taken an overdose of pain pills, but it hadn't worked as he'd hoped. He told the friend, "You'd think 19 pills would've done the job for a guy with a bad ticker like me."

"Even in this moment," Alexa reflects, "he was being totally irreverent, just cutting up."

The friend called Alexa after leaving Alex's home. She told Alexa she feared he would make another attempt to cause his own death, and she asked what she should do.

Alexa told her, "We have to let him do whatever he's going to do. I just don't see a real alternative."

So, the friend left. Alexa and her husband let eight hours go by. Then they went to Alex's home, where they found him alive. But he had indeed made another attempt to end his life. He'd tried this time to cut his wrists, but he was very elderly and the Parkinson's made his movements weak and shaky, and he hadn't been able to manage it.

"We helped him have something to eat and I got him into bed," Alexa says. "For years my father had kept a gun in his nightstand drawer and of course we all knew it was there." Before leaving for the night, Alexa told her dad she was on his side, no matter what, and that she loved him deeply.

Again, Alexa and her husband went home and waited until the next morning. Then they went back and found him dead, as they expected they might.

"You know," Alexa says, "people tell me this story is horrific. They use big loaded words like *horrific*, and I understand why they use those words. My dad was a planner, right? So, he tried Plan A, and then Plan B, and finally he succeeded with Plan C. And Plan C was worse than Plan A, there's no doubt about that.

"But his actual death was not his worst nightmare, and it was not his second-worst nightmare either. And for these reasons, I will not call it horrific. I'll call it heroic! I'll call it self-determined! I'll call it free-thinking and independent! But I won't call it horrific, because from his perspective, it wasn't."

Alexa recalls that her father raised her by himself, and they had a housekeeper to clean and cook meals. This housekeeper developed cancer when Alexa was about twelve. She feared dying in pain and sought Alex's advice on how to avoid that. In response, Alex wrote her a letter that included this paragraph, in which he stated one of his lifelong and deeply held beliefs:

> There is a right to death with dignity which every person should have and which no government should have and which no government or organization can take away. Hard as it is to discuss, I think you are wise to bring the matter up now, so that you can consider it fully. My understanding is that, at this time, there is no official way that anything can be done. It is possible,

of course, to sound out one's doctor on this matter. If he is as wise as you are, he will assure you that he won't let the pain get too great. If he is not so intelligent, he might not. It is important to ask him now.

Alexa was deeply impressed by this piece of correspondence and the fact that Alex had saved it for decades.

"My father was not one to save a copious amount of personal mail," she says, "but he saved this. It was one of very few pieces of correspondence that he saved, and it was prominent among his personal effects when I went through them."

When I think of Alexa's story, I am struck by her love for her father and the fact that her love was great enough to accept his decision to depart this world based on his own well-thought-out principles. But how I wish the Frasers had faced these very important matters in collaboration with a physician willing to speak openly about Alex's desire to advance the time of his death. How I wish his doctor had helped devise a plan to set this as a priority of his healthcare, and plan to invite a death that was both peaceful and affirming of Alex's personhood and dignity.

No elderly and debilitated man should feel forced to saw ineffectually at his wrists with a blade. No devoted daughter should have to agonize about whether he'll successfully carry out his plan while trying to provide him with the space and privacy to do so. Nor should any loving daughter have to enter her father's house to face the aftermath of a death by gunshot. The fact that people feel they must resort to such desperate measures is deplorable and barbaric.

An Ethical Doctrine That Needs to Be Updated

Like Alex Fraser, most people are less afraid of death than of the suffering and deterioration that comes before. They don't want to suffer needlessly while dying. They don't want treatments that merely extend their agony, with no ultimate benefit. Since 1995, the medical community has spent hundreds of millions of dollars to establish and promote the new medical practice known as palliative care. The rise of palliative care represents an enormous advance, in both the philosophy and practice of medicine. But even today, it offers too little to people like Alex Fraser.

The medical system, and palliative care in particular, fails people like Alex Fraser, in part because it is stuck in an old ethical paradigm where hoping to die in order to escape ruthless, relentless deterioration, and then moving with an intention to facilitate death, is openly allowed only in states where the law authorizes medical aid in dying.

This prohibition stifles candid communication and consigns suffering patients to a place of isolation and abandonment.

Here's how this ethical doctrine came about:

In the Middle Ages, St. Thomas Aquinas allowed exceptions to God's commandment not to murder by making "intention" paramount and formulating a "doctrine of double effect." The doctrine absolves a person from responsibility for a death if the person's intention was some other "acceptable" outcome such as the relief of suffering. Under the doctrine, hospice and other palliative care professionals mercifully deliver the large doses of opiates dying patients often require for relief of pain and other symptoms, even though they understand the drugs may hasten death. But the nurses delivering the medication learn to reason that they don't "intend" death. The doctrine also covers a technique called terminal (or palliative) sedation, which means rendering patients unconscious and withholding water and nutrients. The double-effect doctrine enables much of the most merciful end-of-life care we currently have, and we're all grateful for that.

But the prohibition of any responsibility for enabling a timely death at a patient's request stifles candid conversation. The prohibition fails patients, and fails miserably, when it meets the moral framework of a person like Alex. For him, taking responsibility lay at the very core of his moral construct. His life was about standing tall in the face of whatever adversity came to him, making the best plan he could and carrying it out of his own volition.

Everything meaningful to him in his life was over, his suffering was great, his body was useless to him and he was done with it. He wanted to face that and act as responsibly as he knew how.

Maybe Alex tried to talk with his doctor about being ready to die, and maybe the doctor responded in knee-jerk fashion about how helping Alex get his wish would be unethical or illegal. Maybe Alex sensed this would be the doctor's response and did not even try. Either way, it's a shame Alex felt compelled to spurn medical assistance and resort to violent action.

The medical abandonment of Alex Fraser represents a serious deficiency in the rules of bioethics that guide health care professionals. For medicine to remain relevant and helpful, the rules must change. We, the consumers of healthcare, must press for that change.

We need an ethical doctrine to stand in balance with the doctrine of double effect. We need something like a "doctrine of ethical intention," to validate the beliefs of one who would choose to bring their own life to a sensible, rational, intentional and merciful close when pain and other cruel visitations have made living unbearable.

The fact is that every day doctors do things that carry the certain and foreseeable outcome of death. They disconnect ventilators, disable pacemakers, administer terminal sedation and withhold nutrition and hydration. These actions do facilitate death. Clinging to the thought that you don't intend—even a little bit—to bring about the result that is a 100 percent certain outcome of your action must require exhausting mental gymnastics. No wonder doctors and nurses who treat the very sick report high stress levels.

Alex Fraser would never have bothered to try and fit his intention into the moral framework of St. Thomas. He wouldn't have seen any merit in trying. To go a step further, I don't think a keenly moral being could or should try to separate their "intentions" from their foreknowledge of the certain outcome of their actions. If we know a consequence is certain to follow from the action we've decided to take, then we certainly do intend that consequence, otherwise we would not take that action. To pretend otherwise is just plain crazy-making, and it severs any authentic connection between our deep internal clarity and the actions of our daily lives. I've often wondered whether the rigid and convoluted doctrine of double effect contributes to doctors' burnout and the emotional distance so many keep between themselves and their dying patients.

For me, the higher moral ground is occupied by those healthcare workers who acknowledge that some suffering patients *do* want to invite death and their requests, such as to stop renal dialysis or deactivate a cardiac device, arise from that intention. I respect those who accept the grave responsibility of standing with their patient as they invite death.

A moral and authentic actor can accept the burden of responsibility for enabling an intended death, knowing it is rarely justified, and then only under compelling circumstances including the patient's own expressed wish, grievous suffering, a loving family's understanding and support and the imminence of death in any case.

Indeed, the double-effect doctrine serves more as religious doctrinal instruction than ethical guidance, and to me it has always seemed odd to see it so inflexibly enshrined in American law and biomedical ethics.

The system cannot change the system. Only consumers can change the system. Patients who ask questions, make careful decisions and put their own values and priorities first when time is running out: It is they and their loved ones who will change the system.

You who are reading this book are likely to become part of this consumer-driven movement. Through future conversations—conversations with family, doctors, clergy—you and others will construct a new model that no longer produces the kind of desperation Alex Fraser experienced. Regular people with no particular medical training will make the end of life a human, family-centered experience again, just as they brought childbirth out of medical isolation and back to the family. This is our job and is perhaps the last personal, human liberty battle of the baby boom generation and its intrepid descendants.

Choosing a Good Death

The story of Carolyn George begins much like Alex Fraser's. But thanks to a candid, caring, humble and courageous doctor, it ends very differently.

Carolyn George was 81-years-old when she became afflicted with a neuromuscular disease much like ALS or Lou Gehrig's disease. Her condition quickly rendered her weak and debilitated, unable to speak, swallow or move through her home without a walker.

What a drastic change from her former life! Carolyn George had been a celebrated dancer, on Broadway and in the hallowed ranks of the New York City Ballet. Her husband, legendary ballet star Jacques d'Amboise, described her as happiest when she was in the air. She was the very essence of physical vitality—effervescent, graceful, famous for gravity-defying leaps where she seemed to levitate. Is it any wonder, then, that a life utterly devoid of joyful bodily expression felt, to her, without purpose or meaning? Who could say she was wrong to decide not to extend it indefinitely? When the hardships of her compromised life began to outweigh the redemptive aspects, she began to plan her departure.

"My wife had been prescribed pills that would allow her to sleep," d'Amboise recalls. "So, for a while, unbeknownst to anyone in our family, she would take half of each pill every night, and she saved the other half. And then eventually she tried to swallow enough to end her life. But here was the problem: One of the symptoms of her affliction was great difficulty in swallowing. It could take her half an hour to swallow a single pill. So, she fell asleep after taking several of them, before she had taken enough to kill her."

Her unsuspecting husband came home that day to find her collapsed on the floor with the bottle of pills beside her. In his shock and panic, he called 911, thus enrolling her in a medical system that reacted as though she were mentally ill, a pathological danger to herself.

248

D'Amboise continued, "They took her to the hospital and they pumped out her stomach and then they transferred her to the psych ward. And they wouldn't let her out. She was trapped there. It seemed I would need to file a formal petition with a judge and he would have to hear her case and order her release, and that would have taken weeks and weeks.

"It was our good fortune that one of the psychiatric nurses learned the story, because she put us in touch with Compassion & Choices. Through them, I met Dr. David Muller. The only way my wife could get out of the psych ward was to be released into the formal care of a physician. Dr. Muller took on that role and because of him, she was finally able to come home. To this day I am so deeply grateful to him for that. I think of him as a saint." Tears of gratitude fill Jacques' eyes when he comes to Dr. Muller's part of the story.

Indeed, I think of Dr. David Muller as something of a saint, too. He is both learned and kind, humble and capable, funny and wise. I first learned about him on TV, when he spoke frankly on the *Frontline* show I mentioned in the "The Secret of Slow Medicine" chapter. He said some of his patients held a rational desire to end their lives and he felt a duty to help them find a peaceful and legal way to do that. He spoke from vast experience as the Dean for Medical Education at Mount Sinai School of Medicine in New York, and founder and director of its groundbreaking Visiting Doctor Program.

Despite being an Orthodox Jew, Dr. Muller was clear that he would choose the very same outcome for himself because of all that he had learned from his patients and their families during the course of his practice.

He is one of those rare and precious physicians who consider it their job to cure when possible, care always and use his tools and knowledge to help his patients live their best lives and follow their own conscience. Muller served on the board of Compassion & Choices for three years, during which he helped shape the vision and mission that guide us today.

With Dr. Muller taking over Carolyn George's medical care, she came home, relieved, embarrassed and yet no less determined to face the end of her life on her own terms. Dr. Muller remained non-judgmental about her desire. He helped her fashion a plan to accelerate her departure, treat any symptoms or discomfort she might experience and keep her family close throughout the entire process.

With this plan in place, everyone gathered in the family home to celebrate the birthday of one of the sons. By this time, Carolyn had lost any ability to speak. So, toward the end of the party, she shakily penciled a message to her beloved family members.

Jacques remembers, "Carrie said, 'Tomorrow I don't eat or drink, and, before, I want to kiss your eyes.' Then she went around the table, and instead of kissing our tear-filled eyes, she handed us tissues, and giggled."

After looking deeply and lovingly into her family's eyes, she retired to the bedroom and lay down on the bed.

"Everyone was crying," Jacques says. "Our twin daughters didn't go home. They went into the bedroom and lay down on either side of her and softly they talked to her and sang to her and stayed with her for the four or five days it took for her to pass. Most of the rest of the family stayed too. They prepared meals, camped out on the living room floor and reminisced about family history."

Jacques continues, "Dr. Muller was absolutely wonderful. He checked on her continuously. And he told us that after a day or two, he could give her a morphine patch to keep her comfortable. The protocol is not to provide a patch right away, because the idea was that she might change her mind but be too drugged to call it off. But after a certain point, it would be assumed that she did not wish to change her mind and the patch could make her final days much easier."

Jacques was in the next room when his beloved quietly slipped away. The girls were on the bed with her, and they were singing tunes from the Wizard of Oz. One looked down at the end of a song and gasped, "She's gone!"

So gentle was Carolyn's passing, so loving was her care, so sweet and poignant are the memories. Why would any compassionate professional begrudge this woman her intended, planned and self-determined death?

I am truly honored and gratified that our organization was able to play a part in the good ending to Carolyn George's story. Everyone in Carolyn's position, or Alex Fraser's, deserves Dr. Muller's brand of candid expertise and unwavering support.

Navigating the final stages of a progressive illness like ALS, Parkinson's, emphysema, cancer or heart disease is hard. Hard choices come up. Decisions must be made. Everyone should know this: Navigation like this is likely in your future, either on behalf of a loved one or for yourself. To be successful, we need to learn to reveal our hopes and fears, ask important questions and expect candid answers from our healthcare providers. At first this may seem too difficult. But like a muscle, exercise will strengthen our ability to do it. We must start early, years before a medical crisis occurs. You can find a good starter list of tools in the "Tools to Take Charge" appendix following this chapter.

Letting a Disease Take Its Course

These same principles apply to people who are resigned to letting their disease take its course and who simply wish to avoid taking any artificial measures to prolong their lives. These people, however, often face a separate set of challenges in a system set up to relentlessly fight the inevitable.

Testimonies from people with a loved one in this kind of limbo are painfully similar:

> "Three years ago, my mother suffered a massive stroke that left her with serious cognitive impairments. My siblings and I don't think she knows who we are or even who she herself is. She's been bedridden all this time, with a breathing tube and feeding tube. My brothers

share my feeling that enough is enough. Mom would not have wanted to go on this way. But our oldest sister is her medical proxy and she wants to keep the life support. What can we do?" —*Elena R.*

"I'm just grief-stricken over what's happening with my dad. He's in his eighties, with lung cancer, diabetes and kidney disease. He's been in the ICU for weeks. His kidneys are failing, and he can barely breathe on his own. The rest of my family wants the doctors to intubate him and put him on dialysis! There is no way he will ever recover or resume any semblance of his former life, and all these measures will just prolong his misery."

—*Graham S.*

"I can't believe what my brother has gone through and is still going through. After his diagnosis of advanced leukemia, he underwent round after round of painful, debilitating chemo. Now he's in the ICU and all his organs are failing: heart, liver, kidneys. I have begged his wife and grown kids to let him have some peace before he dies. They have got him on every kind of artificial support you can think of and they are still holding out hope for a cure. It's almost like they're colluding in this mass delusion. It's making me furious and it's breaking my heart." —*Ashleigh W.*

Once scenarios like these are in full swing, little can be done to avert needless suffering and mitigate the damage. The key to avoiding such situations in our own lives is to be aware of the looming threat they pose and strengthen the decision-making muscles that will deflect them. Science is on your side. The Institute of Medicine, the American Society of Clinical Oncology, and numerous other researchers and authorities agree that relentless medical aggression hurts patients. It imposes needless suffering on the dying. It is unlikely to extend life and may even shorten it.

Unbelievably, twenty years and hundreds of millions of dollars in medical education and palliative care initiatives have had little impact on such heedless intensive intervention. One in four patients who enter the ICU with documented DNR orders get CPR anyway. Three out of four patients dying of cancer receive last-ditch treatments even the professional oncology society recognizes as harmful. And three in four younger cancer patients with a documented preference for comfort care get at least one aggressive intervention during their last month of life.

This overtreatment exists for a variety of reasons, as I explored in Chapter 3. For instance, some doctors can't bear to tell a dying person when there is no more to be gained from chemotherapy. Some believe that once artificial life support has begun, only the patient's total collapse warrants removing it. Some even believe dying patients owe it to the science of medicine and to society to accept even the most devastating, unproven treatments right up until death, on the remote chance that by "pushing the envelope" something might be learned.

Doctors' motivations, however, are essentially irrelevant when our lives, our values and our priorities for our last precious months are at stake. This is the fundamental difference between medicine's past and its future; the old patterns of paternalism and the future of patient-directedness; the past of "doctor knows best" and the future of truly informed consent to the tests and treatments we undergo.

In a better future, the individuals affected, not their doctors, will align their own values and priorities and decide whether any offered treatment carries a sufficient benefit, or merely imposes a burden too great to accept. Many individuals may still endure low-yield or experimental treatments. But they will do so from altruism and a desire to advance science, not from an expectation of cure for themselves.

You, readers, are the vanguard of an emerging consumer-driven movement. You are the ones who will be mindful, deliberate and who will find your own clarity. You will articulate it to your loved ones, formalize it in writing and above all, let it be your ever-present guide. You will lead with your own determination to live full, joyous and meaningful lives as long as possible, submitting only to those treatment plans that serve your own goals.

It's not always easy to stay true to your own vision. Everything about our current system is designed to resist patient agency. It can be hard to achieve the ending you want—harder than you think. But by building a community of courage, clarity and candor, we can do it.

I began this book with a reflection on the remarkable legacy of those now entering their seventh, eighth and ninth decades. I can't imagine a better way for that legacy to culminate than with a call to reclaim authority over our lives as we age and decline in strength and health. We deserve a home stretch that's in keeping with the lives we've led. We can ensure that the final phase of our lives reflects and upholds the values we cherish and the beliefs we hold.

So, I'll conclude with the same invitation extended in this book's first few pages—an invitation to join the movement for autonomy over how we live as we age.

Let us remain conscious and aware on our ultimate and vital journey.

Let us finish as strong as we've lived.

Tools to Take Charge

Our society is experiencing a profound demographic shift. Every day, 10,000 people turn 65. By 2030, 72 million people will be 65 years or older. As baby boomers reach retirement age, they are becoming the largest generation of people over age 65 in history. Most boomers, like other Americans, want to die at home with loved ones close by, not tethered to machines in the cold isolation of an acute care hospital. But one out of every five U.S. adults will die in the ICU—because intense technology remains the signature of a healthcare system that views death as a failure.

Medicine is a large, entrenched and bureaucratic system, and such systems do not change themselves. Invariably, change comes from outside pressure on the system, and changing expectations in the system. We will transform end-of-life care only when millions of people expect and insist upon something different. We the patients, the people who seek medical treatment, need to create a culture that encourages frank conversations between patients, their loved ones and their doctors about care and choice. Candid conversations will, in turn, help millions of Americans avoid unnecessary suffering in the last stages of illness.

Until we can enact the much-hoped-for transformation in end-of-life care, Compassion & Choices has stepped in to offer a number of hands-on tools designed to build trust, foster candor about the pros and cons of tests and treatments, and to help people assert their own values and priorities as they consent to treatment and make health care decisions. These tools can help people maintain the highest quality of life possible, as illness progresses and their physical condition deteriorates.

For helpful information about advanced planning and the most up-to-date resources, visit CompassionAndChoices.org/endoflifeplanning to find:

Advance Planning Guide

- Getting Started: What Matters Most to You?
- Putting Priorities on Paper: Your Advance Directive
- What I Want: Decisions About Life-Sustaining Measures
- What I Want: Other Documents That Spell Out Choices
- Who Will Speak For Me: Choosing a Representative
- Putting Plans Into Practice:
  Ensuring that Medical Providers Honor Your Wishes
- The Best Safeguard: A Continuing Conversation

Advance Planning Toolkit

- Planning Checklist
- Values Worksheet
- My Particular Wishes for Therapies That Could Sustain Life
- Dementia Provision
- End-of-Life Wishes Letter to Medical Providers
- Sectarian Healthcare Directive
- Rider to Residential Agreement With Assisted-Living Facility
- Hospital Visitation Authorization

About Finish Strong

Finish Strong is an initiative founded by Compassion & Choices to give people with life-threatening illnesses the support, opportunity and courage to live life to the fullest even as illness advances. Compassion & Choices is igniting a social movement that will empower and educate people so they can make fully informed healthcare choices and live their remaining time on their own terms—transforming our health system for all who follow. CompassionAndChoices.org/finish-strong-tools offers interactive tools to use before your doctor's visit: The Trust Card and the Diagnosis Decoder.

The Trust Card is an online service that creates a tool to build strong communication between you and your doctor. Everyone believes their doctor's time is scarce. In an initial visit, patients aren't usually invited to share the values they hope will be honored in the course of their health care. Imagine taking the opportunity in the first few minutes of your medical appointment to set the tone of your relationship with your doctor with the gift of a simple greeting card. The Trust Card enables people to do just that. Find the tool at TrustCard.org.

The Diagnosis Decoder is another online tool to help you ask better questions, so you can receive clearer information and make fully informed treatment decisions. When you visit the Diagnosis Decoder website, you are asked a few questions about your next doctor's appointment. Based on the purpose of the appointment and your concerns, the tool then provides specific questions to ask your doctor, nurse or other health provider—questions designed to get you the complete information you deserve. Visit DiagnosisDecoder.org and learn how to ask the right questions.

Acknowledgments

This book was a long time in the making—a lifetime actually. It would be impossible to name every person along my life and career who informed and inspired my words. But I do want to acknowledge the specific people who helped bring this book from idea to reality.

First, I want to thank Clare Simons and Jason Renaud, who inspired me to write this book. Clare combed through decades of articles, blogs, speeches and interviews and arranged their content into something coherent. She revealed underlying principles and recurrent themes I didn't know were there. Jason doggedly found ways to fit writing into days filled with leading Compassion & Choices and never settled for "no time," as an excuse.

Writer Elissa Karen Wald spent countless hours interviewing me and many of the people profiled in this book. She transcribed many stories and prepared the first draft of most chapters. Her careful attention to detail and skillful writing brought these stories to life.

Editor/project manager Laura E. Kelly read the manuscript at what seemed like its darkest hour and brought it to the light. Or rather, she shone her light of knowledge, experience, and enthusiasm on it, and illuminated the riches that had been buried. From there, Laura became a true book shepherd on *Finish Strong*, cheering me on, guiding me in editing, revising and rearranging the chapters, managing a freelance editorial team (including copyeditor Hannah Billingsley), and overseeing many other crucial aspects of launching this book. My thanks also go to talented book designer Jaye Medalia, who created an elegant and reader-friendly book design, while managing all the many, ever-changing production components with a can-do attitude and good humor.

I learned on this project that it takes a village to publish a book, and I'd like to thank my Compassion & Choices village, whose organization-wide support means so much to me. Writing of the book spanned the tenure of two board chairs, Nancy Hoyt and David Cook. They and the entire board of directors has encouraged and generously supported me throughout.

Kim Callinan, Compassion & Choices CEO, took time out of her very busy schedule to read the manuscript—twice! Kim became its most enthusiastic promoter and I am very grateful to her for believing in the book's power to help people and for dedicating precious resources to make *Finish Strong* available. Kim's editorial suggestions were also invaluable, and made the book richer and more timely. She even contributed her essay about lessons learned from her grandmother's death and the unfortunate limitations of an advance directive.

Bonnie Lawhorn, C&C's national director of marketing and communications, was also an early reader and, as an author herself, jumped into the role of internal point person for this book project. Bonnie coordinated the many C&C resources it took to finalize and launch this book. Those resources included volunteers Kate Ahlport and Doris Fischer whom Executive Volunteer Program Manager, Sarah Brownstein, found to help us take on the laborious job of gathering and organizing permissions and endnote sources.

C&C Senior Design Director Bhavna Kumar brought her special brand of creativity and clarity to develop an evocative and upbeat cover for *Finish Strong*.

As for the book promotion team, Compassion & Choices' Senior National Media Relations Director Sean Crowley, Digital Strategy Director Tracy Rohrbach, Chief Development Officer Linda Roth Platt, Communications Coordinator Alyson Lynch and Direct

Marketing Manager Jane Sanders and their staffs, in particular, went above and beyond in participating in multiple brainstorming sessions and activities to plan a great debut for this book. I am also grateful for the support of the senior program leaders Kim Taccini, Kevin Diaz, Kat West and Charmaine Manansala and their staffs, who have all embraced *Finish Strong* and found creative ways to use it to enhance their own work.

I could never hope to mention all the people by name who contributed to my medical, legal, and advocacy journey. Nevertheless, I would like to extend heartfelt thanks to those who have been my patients and honored me with their trust and openness; those who knew much more about medicine, law, religion, organizations, policy and politics than I did and mentored me through the years; those colleagues who knew how to grow a movement for end-of-life autonomy and dedicated themselves to the task; the many volunteers who have devoted extraordinary energy and countless hours to our work; those who so generously shared their stories, hopes and fears with me and with the world to touch hearts and change minds; those who spent precious and dwindling energy at the close of their lives to make a better experience for those who follow; and those who have supported me and each other with affection and good humor as we labored.

Finally, you read in this book about the important roles played by my parents and sister. But I'd like to acknowledge others in my immediate family, who give my life its joy and meaning: my dear husband, Stephen Lee, and our grown children and their children, who fill me with gratitude for the full-table lives and abundance of love we share.

Notes on Sources

Foreword

page ix   **I was researching my 2017 book *Modern Death* ...** Haider Warraich, *Modern Death: How Medicine Changed the End of Life* (New
York: St. Martin's Press, 2017).

Preface

page xv   **Her son, John F. Kennedy, Jr., emerged from her apartment ...** From video footage on YouTube. https://www.youtube.com/
watch?v=XvqOCSRH4-E. Posted September 6, 2015.

Chapter 1: An Invitation

page 13   **A staggering 85 percent ...** Shereen Jegtvig, "For elderly hospital
patients, CPR often has poor outcome: study," *Reuters*, May 9, 2014,
https://www.reuters.com/article/us-cpr-survival-elderly/for-elderly-
hospital-patients-cpr-often-has-poor-outcome-study-idUSKBN0D-
P1IH20140509.

page 13   **survive resuscitation attempts in the 0 to 2 percent range ...**
"CPR/DNR: A Guide for Family Members," Tri-County Regional Ethics
Committee, September 13, 2016, http://njtrec.org/cprdnr-a-guide-for-
family-members/.

page 13   **Cardiac arrests outside the hospital ...** Berglind Libungan et al.,
"Out-of-hospital cardiac arrest in the elderly: A large-scale population-
based study," *Resuscitation* 94 (September 2015): 28-32, https://doi.
org/.1016/j.resuscitation.2015.05.031.

page 13   **the family of Lorraine Bayless did not take issue ...** Judith
Graham, "Amid CPR Controversy, Many Unanswered Questions,"
New York Times, March 6, 2013, https://newoldage.blogs.nytimes.
com/2013/03/06/amid-cpr-controversy-many-unanswered-questions/?_
r=0.

page 14   **As physician and author Atul Gawande writes ...** Atul Gawande,
Being Mortal: Medicine and What Matters in the End (New York: Met-
ropolitan Books, 2014).

page 20   **As the renowned constitutional scholar, Ronald Dworkin, has
written ...** Ronald Dworkin, *Life's Dominion: An Argument About
Abortion, Euthanasia and Individual Freedom* (New York: Vintage,
1994).

Chapter 2: Talking About Death Won't Kill You (But It Could Improve Your Life)

page 21   **"Do not go gentle into that good night"** ... Poem by Dylan Thomas, from *The Poems of Dylan Thomas*, copyright ©1952 by Dylan Thomas. Reprinted by permission of New Directions Publishing Corp.

page 26   **One large and multi-institutional study was published** ... Baohui Zhang et al., "Health Care Costs in the Last Week of Life: Associations with End of Life Conversations," *Archives of Internal Medicine* 9 (March 2009), https://doi.org/10.1001/archinternmed.2008.587.

page 27   **A second study of 323 cancer patients** ... Alexi A. Wright et al., "Associations Between End-of-Life Discussions, Patient Mental Health, Medical Care Near Death, and Caregiver Bereavement Adjustment," *Journal of the American Medical Association*, 300, no. 14 (October 2008): p. 1665-1673, https://doi.org/10.1001/jama.300.14.1665. https://jamanetwork.com/journals/jama/fullarticle/182700.

page 28   **As Blumenauer put it** ... Earl Blumenauer, "Stop Distorting the Truth about End of Life Care," *HuffPost*, August 24, 2009, http://www.huffingtonpost.com/rep-earl-blumenauer/stop-distorting-the-truth_b_244382.html.

page 28   **In a 2009 radio interview** ... Catharine Richert, "McCaughey claims end-of-life counseling will be required for Medicare patients," POLITIFACT, July 23, 2009, https://www.politifact.com/truth-o-meter/statements/2009/jul/23/betsy-mccaughey/mccaughey-claims-end-life-counseling-will-be-requi/.

page 28   **"Mandatory counseling for all seniors"** ... Ibid.

page 29   **"The America I know and love is not one in which my parents or my baby with Down Syndrome will have to stand in front of Obama's 'death panel'"** ... Brendan Nyhan, "Why the 'Death Panel' Myth Wouldn't Die: Misinformation in the Health Care Reform Debate," *The Forum* 8, issue 1 (2010): 10, https://www.dartmouth.edu/~nyhan/health-care-misinformation.pdf.

page 29   **Jim Dau, a spokesman for the AARP, reported that** ... Jim Dau, "AARP Spokesman on End-of-Life Provision," interview by Robert Siegel, *All Things Considered*, NPR, July 29, 2009, https://www.npr.org/templates/story/story.php?storyId=111341716.

page 29   **In 2014, the Institute of Medicine (IOM) vindicated Blumenauer** ... Institute of Medicine, *Dying in America: Improving Quality and Honoring Individual Preferences Near the End of Life* (Washington, DC: The National Academies Press, 2015), https://doi.org/10.17226/18748.

page 39   **Crows artwork** by David Vandervoort, reprinted with artist's permission, 2018. https://www.davidvandervoort.com/

page 44   **one particular advance directive form called "Five Wishes"** ... "Five Wishes," Five Wishes, https://fivewishes.org/shop/order/product/five-wishes.

Chapter 3: Overtreatment and Diminishing Returns

page 51   **the United States National Academy of Sciences estimated back in 2005 that** ... National Academy of Engineering and Institute of Medicine, *Building a Better Delivery System: A New Engineering/Health Care Partnership*, (Washington, DC: The National Academies Press, 2005), https://doi.org/10.17226/11378.

page 51   **Some estimate up to 30 percent of medical treatment is unnec-
            essary ...** Brendan M. Reilly and Arthur T. Evans, "Much ado about
            (doing) nothing," *Annals of Internal Medicine* 150, no. 4 (February 17,
            2009): p. 270-1, https://doi.org/10.7326/0003-4819-150-4-200902170-
            00008.

page 52   **Dr. Leana Wen, a co-author of the 2014 book *When Doctors
            Don't Listen: How to Avoid Misdiagnoses and Unnecessary Tests*,
            points out that ...** Leana Wen and Joshua Kosowsky, *When Doctors
            Don't Listen: How to Avoid Misdiagnoses and Unnecessary Tests* (New
            York: Thomas Dunne Books, 2013).

page 53   **A final downside of our fee-for-service model ...** The info in this
            paragraph comes from the following sources: Juliet Mavromatis, "Why
            Doctors Interrupt," *The Health Care Blog*, June 12, 2012, http://the-
            healthcareblog.com/blog/2012/06/12/why-doctors-interrupt/. Howard B.
            Beckman and Richard M. Frankel, "The effect of physician behavior on
            the collection of data," *Annals of Internal Medicine* 101, no. 5 (Novem-
            ber 1, 1984): 692-696, https://doi.org/10.7326/0003-4819-101-5-692.
            Donna R. Rhoades et al., "Speaking and interruptions during primary
            care office visits," *Family Medicine* 33, issue 7 (July-August 2001): p.
            528-532, http://www.stfm.org/Portals/49/Documents/FMPDF/Family-
            MedicineVol33Issue7Rhoades528.pdf.

page 55   **she conducted a study to determine whether the grief felt by
            oncologists affected their personal and professional lives ...**
            Leeat Granek et al., "Nature and Impact of Grief Over Patient Loss
            on Oncologists' Personal and Professional Lives," *Archives of Internal
            Medicine* 172, no. 12 (2012): p. 964-966, https://doi.org/10.1001/archin-
            ternmed.2012.1426.

page 55   **Dr. Granek found that ...** Leeat Granek, "When Doctors Grieve," *The
            New York* Times, May 25, 2012, https://www.nytimes.com/2012/05/27/
            opinion/sunday/when-doctors-grieve.html.

page 55   **She explains that both doctors and patients benefit ...** Danielle
            Ofri, *What Doctors Feel: How Emotions Affect the Practice of Medicine*
            (Boston: Beacon Press, 2014).

page 56   **Suppressed grief threatens mental health ...** Jessica Berthold,
            "The emotional life of doctors," *ACP Hospitalist*, November 2013,
            https://acphospitalist.org/archives/2013/11/qa.htm.

page 56   **A growing number of programs, from those at the University of
            California in Los Angeles to others at Mount Sinai in New York
            ...** Lucette Lagnado, "Training Doctors to Manage Their Feelings," *Wall
            Street Journal*, May 9, 2016, https://www.wsj.com/articles/training-
            doctors-to-manage-their-feelings-1462808283.

page 57   **Dr. Ken Murray, a retired family practice physician ...** Ken
            Murray, "How Doctors Die," *Zocalo Public Square*, November 30, 2011,
            http://www.zocalopublicsquare.org/2011/11/30/how-doctors-die/ideas/
            nexus.

page 58   **"I would like to say, 'Family, only you can..."** David S. Pisetsky,
            "Doing Everything," *Annals of Internal Medicine* 128, no. 10 (May 15,
            1998): 869-870, https://doi.org/10.7326/0003-4819-128-10-199805150-
            00013.

page 58   **Every year the researchers at Dartmouth Atlas Project map
            the utilization ...** "The Dartmouth Atlas of Health Care," Dartmouth
            Atlas, 2018, http://www.dartmouthatlas.org/.

page 59   **Dr. Daniel Callahan of The Hastings Center, a research institu-
           tion dedicated to bioethics and the public interest, reports that
           ...** Daniel Callahan, "Health Care Costs and Medical Technology," in
           *From Birth to Death and Bench to Clinic: The Hastings Center Bioethics
           Briefing Book for Journalists, Policymakers, and Campaigns*, ed. Mary
           Crowley (Garrison, NY: The Hastings Center, 2008), p. 79-82, https://
           www.thehastingscenter.org/wp-content/uploads/Health-Care-Costs-
           BB17.pdf.

page 59   **According to a national physicians' survey conducted in 2010
           by Jackson Healthcare ...** "Physician Study: Quantifying the Cost of
           Defensive Medicine," Jackson Healthcare, February 2010, https://jack-
           sonhealthcare.com/media-room/surveys/defensive-medicine-study-2010/.

page 59   **The executives' responses revealed that defensive medicine ...**
           Fred Pennic, "Is Defensive Medicine Driving Up Healthcare Costs?,"
           HIT Consultant, April 10, 2014, https://hitconsultant.net/2014/04/10/is-
           defensive-medicine-driving-up-healthcare-costs/.

page 60   **In August 2010, a study of 151 cancer patients ...** Jennifer S. Temel
           et al., "Early Palliative Care for Patients with Metastatic Non-Small-
           Cell Lung Cancer," *The New England Journal of Medicine* 363, no. 8
           (August 19, 2010): 733-742, https://doi.org/10.1056/NEJMoa1000678.

page 63   **In 2011, the National Journal and the Regence Foundation
           teamed up to survey Americans ...** "Living Well at the End of Life:
           A National Conversation," Interview conducted by *National Journal*,
           2011, http://syndication.nationaljournal.com/communications/National-
           JournalRegenceToplines.pdf.

Chapter 4: Let Me Die Like a Doctor

page 68   **This revelation took the nation by storm in November 2011
           when Dr. Ken Murray ...** Ken Murray, "How Doctors Die," *Zocalo
           Public Square*, November 30, 2011, http://www.zocalopublicsquare.
           org/2011/11/30/how-doctors-die/ideas/nexus/.

page 69   **London's Daily Mail re-printed the article under the provoca-
           tive headline: "Why Most Doctors Like Me Would Rather DIE"
           ...** Martin Scurr, "Why MOST doctors like me would rather DIE than
           endure the pain of treatment we inflict on others for terminal diseases:
           Insider smashes medicine big taboo," *Mail Online*, February 14, 2012,
           http://www.dailymail.co.uk/health/article-2100684/Why-doctors-like-die-
           endure-pain-treatment-advanced-cancer.html.

page 69   **In 2014, Dr. V.J. Periyakoil, the director of the Stanford Pallia-
           tive Care Education and Training Program, conducted a study
           ...** Vyjeyanthi S. Periyakoil et al., "Do Unto Others: Doctors' Personal
           End-of-Life Resuscitation Preferences and Their Attitudes toward
           Advance Directives," PLoS ONE 9, issue 5 (May 2014): https://doi.
           org/10.1371/journal.pone.0098246.

page 70   **In 2016, researchers at the University of Colorado looking at
           treatment patterns in 200,000 Medicare beneficiaries found that
           ...** Daniel D. Matlock et al., "How U.S. Doctors Die: A Cohort Study of
           Healthcare Use at the End of Life," *Journal of the American Geriat-
           rics Society* 64, issue 5 (May 2016): 1061-1067, https://doi.org/10.1111/
           jgs.14112.

page 71   **In his posthumous 2016 memoir *When Breath Becomes Air* ...**
           Excerpts in this section are from *When Breath Becomes Air* by Paul

Kalanithi, copyright © 2015 by Corcovado, Inc. Used by permission of Random House, an imprint and division of Penguin Random House LLC. All rights reserved.

page 72   **On her book tour, his wife Lucy sat down with Katie Couric to discuss** ... Brad Marshland, "'When Breath Becomes Air:' a dying doctor's memoir teaches about love and loss," *Yahoo! News*, January 22, 2016, https://www.yahoo.com/katiecouric/when-breath-becomes-aira-young-father-and-133132815.html?soc_src=mail&soc_trk=ma.

Chapter 5: Hope and Heroism

page 78   **a comment in the press from Bob Dole, now 94** ... Jonathan Martin, "At His Ranch, John McCain Shares Memories and Regrets With Friends," *The New York Times*, May 5, 2018, https://www.nytimes.com/2018/05/05/us/politics/john-mccain-arizona.html.

page 78   **"I wanted to let him know how much I love him"** ... Ibid.

page 78   **"McCain is not just plotting the details of his own funeral but living it"** ... Timothy Egan, "As He Lay Dying," *The New York* Times, May 11, 2018, https://www.nytimes.com/2018/05/11/opinion/john-mccain-trump-funeral-death.html.

page 79   **Not long ago, *The Atlantic* published an article titled "The Trouble With Medicine's Metaphors"** ... Dhruv Khullar, "The Trouble with Medicine's Metaphors," *The Atlantic*, August 7, 2014, https://www.theatlantic.com/health/archive/2014/08/the-trouble-with-medicines-metaphors/374982/.

page 79   **Cancer survivor Heather Lagemann says** ... Kareem Yasin, "Living with Cancer: Am I a Warrior?," *Healthline*, May 26, 2015, https://www.healthline.com/health/cancer/living-with-cancer-warrior#2.

page 80   **Marjorie Williams, writing about her liver cancer in her posthumous 2006 book** ... Marjorie Williams, *The Woman at the Washington Zoo: Writings on Politics, Family and Fate* (New York: PublicAffairs, 2006).

page 81   **In 2014, a 29-year-old woman named Brittany Maynard** ... Brittany's story is retold throughout this book with the kind permission of her husband, Dan Diaz.

page 81   **and he underwent many new and experimental treatments** ... Lindsey Bever, "Every Single Day is a Gift: This dying man openly opposed assisted suicide in his last days," *The Washington Post*, July 25, 2018, https://www.washingtonpost.com/news/to-your-health/wp/2018/07/25/every-single-day-is-a-gift-this-dying-man-openly-opposed-assisted-suicide-in-his-last-days/.

page 82   **Amanda Bennett delivered a TED talk based on her book *The Cost of Hope*** ... Amanda Bennett, "The Cost of Hope," filmed April 2013 at TEDMED 2013, Washington, D.C., video, https://www.ted.com/talks/amanda_bennett_a_heroic_narrative_for_letting_go.

page 84   **In an article for *Bloomberg Businessweek*, she later reflected** ... Amanda Bennett, "Lessons of a $618,616 Death," *Bloomberg Businessweek*, March 5, 2010, https://www.bloomberg.com/news/articles/2010-03-04/lessons-of-a-618-616-death.

page 85   **"The God Abandons Antony"** ... *"The God Abandons Antony,"* C.P. Cavafy, *Collected Poems*. Translated from the Greek by Edmund Keeley and Philip Sherrard. Edited by George Savidis. Revised Edition. Princeton University Press, 1992).

page 85   **"Do not stoop to strategies like this"** ... Leonard Cohen, "Alexandra Leaving," *Ten New Songs*, 2001.

page 86   **American sportscaster, Stuart Scott, offered just such a brave new story** ... "Stuart Scott's 2014 Jimmy V Award Acceptance Speech," YouTube, July 11, 2017, https://www.youtube.com/watch?v=4TdF07xO-eo&feature=youtu.be.

page 86   **"Dying is not the worst thing that can happen to you"** ... Paul Smith, *Facing Death: The Deep Calling to the Deep* (Coat of Many Colors, 1999).

Chapter 6: Hospice: The Healing Option

page 87   **"Would earlier hospice care have been kinder?"** ... Amanda Bennett, "Lessons of a $618,616 Death," *Bloomberg Businessweek*, March 4, 2010.

page 87   **"Drink it in"** ... Leonard Cohen, "Alexandra Leaving," *Ten New Songs*, 2001.

page 88   **Her decision was pointedly made public on April 16** ... Nicole Spector, "Barbara Bush is choosing 'comfort care.' What does it mean? More than you may think," *NBC News*, April 17, 2018, https://www.nbcnews.com/better/health/barbara-bush-choosing-comfort-care-what-does-it-entail-more-you-ncna866596.

page 88   **One of the common myths about palliative care** ... Melissa Bailey and JoNel Aleccia, "Barbara Bush's End-Of-Life Decision Stirs Debate Over 'Comfort Care,'" *Kaiser Health News*, April 16, 2018, https://khn.org/news/barbara-bushs-end-of-life-decision-stirs-debate-over-comfort-care/.

page 88   **Another source close to the Bush family told CBS** ... Julia Birkinbine, "Barbara Bush Spent Her Last Days Surrounded by Her Loved Ones," *Closer*, April 21, 2018, https://www.closerweekly.com/posts/barbara-bush-death-158367.

page 89   **"by bringing this into the sphere of discussion, we can start thinking about comfort and palliation"** ... Melissa Bailey and JoNel Aleccia, "Barbara Bush's End-Of-Life Decision Stirs Debate Over 'Comfort Care,'" *see above.*

page 90   **The Julianna Snow story was assembled from the following sources:** Elizabeth Cohen, "Heaven over hospital: Dying girl, aged 5, makes a choice," (Part 1), CNN, October 27, 2015, https://edition.cnn.com/2015/10/27/health/girl-chooses-heaven-over-hospital-part-1/index.html. Elizabeth Cohen, "Heaven over hospital: Dying girl, aged 5, makes a choice," (Part 2), CNN, November 4, 2015, http://www.cnn.com/2015/10/27/health/girl-chooses-heaven-over-hospital-part-2/. Myriah Towner, 'I'd rather go to heaven than hospital again': Girl, 5, with incurable neurodegenerative disease tells her parents what to do when she gets really sick again," Mail Online, October 28, 2015, https://www.dailymail.co.uk/news/article-3292571/Girl-5-incurable-disease-tells-parents-d-heaven-hospital.html.Michelle Moon, "How Our Daughter Helps Us Face Our Greatest Fear," *The Mighty*, June 1, 2015, https://themighty.com/2015/06/daughter-with-charcot-marie-tooth-disease-embraces-dying/.

page 92   **beginning in the 11ᵗʰ century** ... "A History of Hospice: A Timeline of One of Medicine's Oldest Disciplines," 1-800-HOSPICE, November 20, 2016, https://www.1800hospice.com/end-of-life-care/history-hospice/.

page 92   **Cicely Saunders started the first modern hospice in 1967 ...** "History and Dame Cicely Saunders," St. Christopher's Hospice | London website, http://www.stchristophers.org.uk/about/history.

page 94   **Dr. Ziad Obermeyer, a health policy specialist at Harvard Medical School ...** Ziad Obermeyer et al., "Association Between the Medicare Hospice Benefit and Health Care Utilization and Costs for Patients with Poor-Prognosis Cancer," JAMA 312, no. 18 (November 12, 2014): p. 1886-1896, https://doi.org/10.1001/jama.2014.14950.

page 95   *Health Affairs* **published a study examining the emergency department visits of patients ...** Alexander K. Smith et al., "Half of Older Americans Seen in Emergency Department in Last Month of Life; Most Admitted to Hospital, And Many Die There," *Health Affairs* 31, no. 6 (June 2012), https://doi.org/10.1377/hlthaff.2011.0922.

page 95   **the Medicare Access and CHIP Reauthorization Act of 2015 ...** "H.R.2 - Medicare Access and CHIP Reauthorization Act of 2015," Congress.gov, p. 2015-2016, https://www.congress.gov/bill/114th-congress/house-bill/2.

page 96   **An example of that irrational thinking showed up in a** *60 Minutes II* **segment ...** Dan Rather, "A Question of Homicide? The Diagnosis: Cancer," *CBS News*, June 22, 1999, https://www.cbsnews.com/news/a-question-of-homicide/.

page 97   **Hospital deaths accounted for only 19.8 percent of all deaths ...** "Fewer Medicare beneficiaries dying in the hospital, but ICU use at end-of-life still common," *ACP Hospitalist Weekly*, July 4, 2018, https://acphospitalist.org/weekly/archives/2018/07/04/1.htm.

page 97   **admissions to the ICU during the last 30 days of life are rising ...** Joan Teno, Pedro L. Gozalo, et al. "Change in End-of-Life Care for Medicare Beneficiaries: Site of Death, Place of Care and Health Care Transitions in 2000, 2005 and 2009." JAMA February 6, 2013, Vol 309, No 5, p. 470–477.

page 98   **"Palliative care, and the medical sub-specialty of palliative medicine" ...** "What Is Palliative Care?" Center to Advance Palliative Care, https://www.capc.org/payers-policymakers/what-is-palliative-care/.

page 99   **"It's not our job as health professionals" ...** Bob Tedeschi, "Stop accepting death: A doctor rejects medicine's 'self-righteous' approach with patients," *Stat*, March 13, 2017, https://www.statnews.com/2017/03/13/death-patients-diane-meier/.

page 99   **"You're letting your life be defined by the fear of death" ...** Ibid.

page 99   **If the goal of palliative care is to ...** "About Palliative Care," Center to Advance Palliative Care, https://www.capc.org/about/palliative-care/.

page 100   **which she called "the final stage of growth" ...** Elisabeth Kübler-Ross, *Death: The Final Stage of Growth* (New York: Touchstone, 1986).

page 101   **Drs. Miles J. Edwards and Susan W. Tolle of Oregon Health and Sciences University described an exemplary palliative treatment ...** Miles J. Edwards and Susan W. Tolle, "Disconnecting a Ventilator at the Request of a Patient Who Knows He Will Then Die: A Doctor's Anguish," *Annals of Internal Medicine* 117, no. 3 (August 1, 1992): p. 254-256, https://doi.org/10.7326/0003-4819-117-3-254.

page 102   **"Then came the particularly difficult question" ...** Ibid.

page 104   **"Mr. Larson seemed comfortable" ...** Ibid.

page 104   **"We took turns listening" ...** Ibid.

page 104   **"the harmonizing of the disquieted"** ... Stephen Levine, *Healing into Life and Death* (Knopf Doubleday Publishing Group, 1989), p. 3-4.

page 105   **Stephen's books, including** ... Stephen and Ondrea Levine, *Who Dies? An Investigation of Conscious Living and Conscious Dying* (Anchor Books, 1982).

page 105   **"Quiet completion" and "greater wellness ... their future wide open"** ... Stephen Levine, *Healing into Life and Death* (Knopf Doubleday Publishing Group, 1989), p. 5.

Chapter 7: The Secret of Slow Medicine

page 106   **"Slow medicine"** ... Alberto Delara, "Invitation to 'Slow Medicine,'" *Italian Heart Journal, Supplement: Official Journal of the Italian Journal of Cardiology* 3, no. 1 (January 2002): p. 100-101.

page 108   **Three essential tenets of good care** ... As told to Elissa Karen Wald in an interview for this book.

page 109   **In 2012, the journal *Intensive Care Medicine* published research on the conversations doctors held with** ... Yael Schenker et al., "Association between physicians' beliefs and the option of comfort care for critically ill patients," *Intensive Care Medicine* 38, issue 10 (October 2012): p. 1607-1615.

page 110   **As the editors of *Intensive Care Medicine* wrote** ... Erin K. Kross, "Do physicians' beliefs influence treatment options at the end of life?" *Intensive Care Medicine* 38, issue 10 (October 2012): p. 1586-1587.

page 110   **a *Frontline* documentary featuring patients in a bone marrow transplant unit** ... Miri Navasky and Karen O'Connor, "Facing Death," *Frontline*, November 23, 2010, https://www.pbs.org/wgbh/pages/frontline/facing-death/etc/transcript.html.

page 112   **Palliative Care Information Act** ... New York State, effective February 9, 2011, https://www.health.ny.gov/professionals/patients/patient_rights/palliative_care/information_act.htm.

page 115   **One leading proponent of the slow medicine movement is Dr. Victoria Sweet** ... Victoria Sweet, *God's Hotel: A Doctor, a Hospital, and a Pilgrimage to the Heart of Medicine* (New York: Riverhead Books, 2012) and *Slow Medicine: The Way to Healing* (New York: Riverhead Books, 2017).

page 115   **Interview with Dr. Victoria Sweet** ... "The Efficiency of Inefficiency," Victoria Sweet at TEDxMiddlebury, http://tedxtalks.ted.com/video/The-Efficiency-of-Inefficiency (published August 15, 2013).

page 116   **As Dr. Sweet says in her 2017 book** ... Victoria Sweet, *Slow Medicine: The Way to Healing* (New York: Riverhead Books, 2017), p. 247-268.

page 116   **Rob's story in his own words** ... From an interview conducted by Elissa Karen Wald for this book.

page 123   **speech by Dr. Francis Peabody** ... Dr. Francis W. Peabody, "The Care of the Patient," speech given October 1926; article "The Care of the Patient," *JAMA* 88, no. 12 (1927), https://doi.org/10.1001/jama.1927.02680380001001.

page 123   **Dr. Dennis McCullough** ... Dennis McCullough, *My Mother, Your Mother: Embracing Slow Medicine, the Compassionate Approach to Caring for Your Aging Loved Ones* (New York, HarperCollins Publishers, 2008).

page 125   Jane Kenyon's poem, "Otherwise" ... Jane Kenyon and Donald Hall, *Otherwise: New and Selected Poems* (Graywolf Press, 1996).

page 126   **"Such fears are rarely shared"** ... Jane Gross, "For the Elderly, Being Heard About Life's End," *The New York Times*, May 5, 2008, https://www.nytimes.com/2008/05/05/health/05slow.html.

page 128   **"'Fast Medicine' is running its lockstep, breakneck course"** ... Dennis McCullough, *My Mother, Your Mother: Embracing Slow Medicine, the Compassionate Approach to Caring for Your Aging Loved Ones* (New York, HarperCollins Publishers, 2008).

Chapter 8: Escaping Dementia

page 133   **"she shrieks with fear"** ... Paula Span, "In Elderly Hands, Firearms Can Be Even Deadlier," *The New York Times*, May 25, 2018, https://www.nytimes.com/2018/05/25/health/elderly-guns-suicide-dementia.html.

page 134   **Paula Span documented these dangers** ... Ibid.

page 134   **According to the Alzheimer's Association** ... Facts and Figures, Alzheimer's Association, 2018, https://alz.org/alzheimers-dementia/facts-figures and 2018 Alzheimer's Disease Facts and Figures Infographic, https://alz.org/media/Documents/alzheimers-facts-and-figures-infographic.pdf. Visit the World Health Organization website for updated statistics: http://www.who.int.

page 134   **the "Health and Retirement Study"** ... Kenneth M. Langa et al., "A Comparison of the Prevalence of Dementia in the United States in 2000 and 2012," *JAMA Internal Medicine* 177, no.1 (2017), p. 51-58, https://doi.org/10.1001/jamainternmed.2016.6807.

page 135   **The Alzheimer's Association reports that** ... Alz.org website, https://alz.org/alzheimers-dementia/facts-figures from 2018 and 2014.

page 136   **9 of every 10 people living with dementia** ... BZ Aminoff, A. Adunsky, "Dying dementia patients: too much suffering, too little palliation," Am J Hosp Palliat Care. Sept-Oct 2005; 22(5); p. 344-8.

page 137   **Only 45 percent of Alzheimer's patients (or their caregivers)** ... New Alzheimer's Association report finds less than half of people with Alzheimer's disease say they were told the diagnosis," Alzheimer's Association, March 23, 2015. https://www.alz.org/news/2015/new-alzheimer_s-association-report-finds-less-%284%29.

page 138   **Below are some of those genuine warnings** ... "10 early signs and symptoms of Alzheimer's," Alzheimer's Association, 2018, https://alz.org/alzheimers-dementia/10_signs.

page 142   **Guide to Determine Alzheimer's Disease or Dementia Stages** ... "CBAS Eligibility Determination Tools & Guidance," California Department of Health Care Services, 2018, http://www.dhcs.ca.gov/services/Pages/CBASEligiblityDeterminationToolsGuidance.aspx.

page 150   **I had the privilege of assisting State Senator Robert Shoemaker as he fought to include a dementia provision within the standard advance directive** ... "The Dementia Provision," Compassion & Choices, May 2018, compassionandchoices.org/wp-content/uploads/2018/05/Dementia_Provision1.pdf.

page 159   **The account of [Sandy Bem's] decline and her response to it was featured in *The New York Times Magazine* in May of 2015** ... Robin Marantz Henig, "The Last Day of Her Life," *The New York Times Magazine*, May 14, 2015, https://www.nytimes.com/2015/05/17/magazine/the-last-day-of-her-life.html.

page 160   **Afterward, NPR aired a story about Sandy in which the journal-**

ist Alix Spiegel noted ... Alix Spiegel, "How A Woman's Plan to Kill Herself Helped Her Family Grieve," *NPR*, June 23, 2014, https://www. npr.org/sections/health-shots/2014/06/23/323330486/how-a-womans-plan-to-kill-herself-helped-her-family-grieve.

page 161   **Janet Adkins, the first person to die in the back of Kevork-ian's Volkswagen bus** ... Brian Meehan, "Suicide of Portland's Janet Adkins with Kevorkian's help brings euthanasia issue into spotlight," *The Oregonian / OregonLive*, June 10, 1990, https://www.oregonlive.com/ health/index.ssf/1990/06/portlands_janet_adkins_suicide.html.

page 161   **Ron Adkins sent a heartfelt letter to the Alzheimer's Association** ... Alzheimer's Association Fact Sheet: "Suicide and Assisted Suicide," https://www.theirisproject.net/uploads/7/8/4/1/78413882/alzassoc_sui-cide_and_assisted_suicide.pdf.

page 162   **Gillian documented her final thoughts on her website** ... "Goodbye and Good Luck!" *deadatnoon.com*, August 18, 2014, http://deadat-noon.com/.

Chapter 9: Inside a Growing Advocacy

page 174   **"I've got a lot of things going on in my mind these days because life hasn't gone the way I planned it"** ... "The Last Campaign of Governor Booth Gardner," Vimeo, 2009, https://vimeo.com/9500266.

page 174   **"Prejudice just went right over my head"** ... John C. Hughes, *Booth Who? A Biography of Booth Gardner, Washington's Charismatic Governor* (Washington State Legacy Project, Office of the Secretary of State, 2010), p. 60, https://www.sos.wa.gov/legacy/stories/booth-gardner/ pdf/complete.pdf.

page 175   **Fifteen years later, in a documentary about his last political campaign, he would tell the interviewer** ... "The Last Campaign of Governor Booth Gardner," Vimeo, 2009, https://vimeo.com/9500266.

page 175   **"This is not going to sit well with some of you"** ... Ibid.

page 177   **"I hear a story a day"** ... Ibid.

page 178   **"Please help me keep my promise to my husband"** ... John C. Hughes, *Booth Who? A Biography of Booth Gardner, Washington's Charismatic Governor* (Washington State Legacy Project, Office of the Secretary of State, 2010), p. 174, https://www.sos.wa.gov/legacy/stories/ booth-gardner/pdf/complete.pdf.

page 178   **The actor Martin Sheen shot an opposition ad** ... Ibid., p. 175-176.

page 178   **Barbara Roberts, former governor of Oregon, appeared as the ultimate validator** ... Ibid., 177.

page 179   **"On election night I do not allow myself to get too happy"** ... Ibid., p. 178.

page 180   **"He was so skinny he couldn't sit"** ... Susan Donaldson James, "Daughter Hails Montana's Right-to-Die Ruling," *ABC News*, January 6, 2010, https://abcnews.go.com/Health/doctor-assisted-suicide-approved-montana/story?id=9492923.

page 180   **"Bob approached us and asked if there was anything we could do from a legal standpoint"** ... From personal communication with Barbara Coombs Lee.

page 182   **The most recognizable face of California's multi-year campaign will always be Brittany Maynard** ... "Dying with Dignity (Brittany Maynard)," YouTube, November 28, 2016, https://www.youtube.com/ watch?v=GXgNmHdVRLY.

page 183   **No one can tell her story with more accuracy and immediacy than Patty herself ...** From an interview conducted by Elissa Karen Wald for this book.

page 191   **Recent polls by Gallup and Harris ...** "Polling on Voter Support for Medical Aid in Dying for Terminally Ill Adults," Compassion & Choices, February 2, 2016, https://compassionandchoices.org/resource/polling-medical-aid-dying/.

Chapter 10: People Taking Control

page 198   **One such conversation was with Dr. Kathleen Morris ...** Diane Rehm radio interview with Dr. Morris, "Choosing to Die," WAMU/88.5 radio show, July 7, 2014 https://dianerehm.org/shows/2014-07-07/choosing-die.

page 202   **Reverend Ross tells the story of one such congregant, a young woman named Dawn ...** From an interview conducted with Elissa Karen Wald for this book.

page 206   **"I have to tell you, when you're 29 years old, being told you have that kind of timeline" ...** Quotes throughout this chapter are taken from Compassion & Choices video interviews with Brittany Maynard. "The Brittany Maynard Story," YouTube, October 6, 2014, https://www.youtube.com/watch?v=yPfe3rCcUeQ.

page 209   **"I would not tell anyone else that he or she should" ...** Brittany Maynard, "My right to death with dignity at 29," *CNN*, November 2, 2014, http://edition.cnn.com/2014/10/07/opinion/maynard-assisted-suicide-cancer-dignity/index.html.

Chapter 11: Space for the Sacred

page 215   **The overwhelming majority of Americans worship a supreme spiritual being ...** Frank Newport, "Most Americans Still Believe in God," *Gallup*, June 29, 2016, https://news.gallup.com/poll/193271/americans-believe-god.aspx.

page 215   **"a greater moral deficit than the other states" ...** Barbara Coombs Lee, "On My Mind: Pro-Choice and Pro-God," Compassion in Dying, *The Body*, Fall 2001, http://www.thebody.com/content/art16709.html.

page 216   **"All religions must be tolerated" ...** "Frederick the Great Quotes," AZ Quotes, https://www.azquotes.com/author/5837-Frederick_The_Great.

page 217   **Reverend Madison Shockley... illustrates this with the story of King Saul ...** From a personal interview with Barbara Coombs Lee.

page 218   **Each In his Own Tongue ...** William Herbert Carruth, "Each in His Own Tongue," Representative Poetry Online—Online at University of Toronto Libraries, 2002, https://rpo.library.utoronto.ca/poems/each-his-own-tongue.

page 219   **Reverend Ralph Mero, one of the founders of Compassion in Dying often described God's gift of life as, "More a loan than a gift" ...** Personal correspondence with Barbara Coombs Lee.

page 220   **Char Andrews, a client who helped us defend Oregon's law ...** Barbara Coombs Lee, *Compassion in Dying: Stories of Dignity and Choice* (NewSage Press, 2003).

page 222   ***The Bond Between Women, a Journey to Fierce Compassion ...*** China Galland, *The Bond between Women, a Journey to Fierce Compassion* (Darby: Diane Pub. Co., 1998).

page 226   **"Death," he writes, "is *not* a cosmic mistake." ...** Rabbi Zalman
             Schachter-Shalomi and Ronald S. Miller, *From AGE-ing to Sage-ing:
             A Profound New Vision of Growing Older* (New York: Warner Books,
             1995), 81.
page 227   **Rabbi Zalman and others explain the tasks of life ...** James Hill-
             man, *The Soul's Code: In Search of Character and Calling* (New York:
             Ballantine Books, Reprint edition - August 1, 2017).
page 228   **Spanish poet Antonio Machado captures a wonderful image ...**
             Antonio Machado, *Times Alone: Selected Poems of Antonio Machado*,
             translated by Robert Bly (Middletown, CT: Wesleyan University Press,
             1983), p. 13.
page 228   **As poet Mary Oliver writes, "When will you have a little pity"**
             ... Mary Oliver, *Blue Pastures* (New York: Houghton Mifflin Harcourt
             Publishing Company, 1995), p. 47.
page 228   **Sallirae Henderson writes of the importance ...** Sallirae Hender-
             son, *A Life Complete: Emotional and Spiritual Growth for Midlife and
             Beyond* (New York: Scribner, Simon & Schuster, 2000), p. 26 (Kindle
             version).
page 228   **"Forgiveness work" ...** Rabbi Zalman Schachter-Shalomi and Ronald
             S. Miller, *From AGE-ing to Sage-ing,* see above.
page 229   **South Africa's Truth and Reconciliation Commission ...** "Truth
             and Reconciliation Commission, South Africa," Encyclopaedia Britan-
             nica, https://www.britannica.com/topic/Truth-and-Reconciliation-Com-
             mission-South-Africa.
page 229   **"When they asked to be forgiven" ...** Pieter Hugo (photographs)
             and Susan Dominus, "Portraits of Reconciliation," *The New York
             Times Magazine*, April 6, 2014, https://www.nytimes.com/interac-
             tive/2014/04/06/magazine/06-pieter-hugo-rwanda-portraits.html.
page 229   **"Never again" ...** Samantha Power, "Never Again: The World's Most
             Unfulfilled Promise," Frontline/PBS, https://www.pbs.org/wgbh/pages/
             frontline/shows/karadzic/genocide/neveragain.html.
page 230   **In 2015, about 160,000 Americans had defibrillators implanted ...**
             Sandeep Jauhar, "How Do You Want to Die," *The New York Times*, July
             29, 2018. https://www.nytimes.com/2018/07/28/opinion/sunday/cardiac-
             defibrillator-death.html.
page 231   **As Kathy Black explains in her book of ritual resources for
             women ...** Kathy Black, *Wising Up: Ritual Resources for Women of
             Faith in Their Journey of Aging* (Eugene: Wipf & Stock, 2010).
page 232   **"I'll Fly Away" ...** Albert E. Brumley, (c) Copyright 1932 in "Wonderful
             Message" by Hartford Music Co. Renewed 1960 by Albert E. Brumley &
             Sons/SESAC (admin by ClearBox Rights). All rights reserved. Used by
             permission.

Chapter 12: It's Harder Than You Think (But We Can Do It)

page 240   **"He had gallons of water in his basement in case the water main
             were ever compromised" ...** These stories about Alex Fraser were
             provided in an interview of Alexa Fraser conducted by Elissa Karen
             Wald for this book.
page 248   **Carolyn George was 81 years old when she became afflicted ...**
             These stories about Carolyn George were provided in an interview of
             Jacques d'Amboise conducted by Elissa Karen Wald for this book.
page 253   **One in four patients who enter the ICU with documented**

DNR orders get CPR anyway ... Hart et al. "Variability among US intensive care units in managing the care of patients admitted with preexisting limits on life-sustaining therapies," *JAMA Internal Medicine*, 2015; 175:1019-26, http://archinte.jamanetwork.com/article.aspx?articleid=2210886.

page 253   **Three out of four patients dying of cancer receive last-ditch** ... Chen et al. 2016. "Aggressive care at the end-of-life for younger patients with cancer: Impact of ASCO's Choosing Wisely campaign." *Journal of Clinical Oncology* 34, 2016 (suppl; abstr LBA10033). http://meetinglibrary.asco.org/content/170424-176.

page 253   **And three in four younger cancer patients ...** J Palliat, JW Mack, "Care in the Final Month of Life among Adolescent and Young Adult Cancer Patients in Kaiser Permanente Southern California," Med. 2016 Aug 2, http://www.ncbi.nlm.nih.gov/pubmed/27482745.

About the Author

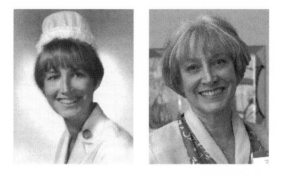

Over more than five decades, Barbara Coombs Lee worked in healthcare as a clinician, policymaker and advocate. Her indelible bedside experiences forged a deep respect for individual values and beliefs and eventually led her to a career in law and health policy. For the last 25 years she has advocated for initiatives that allow individuals a full range of options and much greater agency in their healthcare decisions.

Barbara's work in public policy culminated in her roles as chief executive officer and president of Compassion & Choices, the nation's oldest and largest organization working to empower everyone to chart their end-of-life journey. After serving in this capacity for 22 years, Barbara transitioned her role to President Emerita/Senior Adviser. Thousands of personal experiences and the teachings of scholars and thought leaders around the globe inform her perspective. She is a seasoned writer, speaker and commentator.

Barbara's passion for transforming the end-of-life experience by informing and empowering patients infuses *Finish Strong*. She calls for all Americans to join a patient-driven movement to dismantle the institutional and cultural barriers to living well to the very end.

She lives in Oregon.

About
Compassion & Choices

Compassion & Choices is the nation's oldest, largest and most active nonprofit working to improve care and expand options for the end of life. From our origin in 1980, we have united over 450,000 supporters nationwide to become the preeminent leader of the movement for end-of-life options.

How we live the final chapter of our lives, and how we die, are among our most deeply personal experiences. While in theory, we can decide how much or how little treatment we want, our current healthcare system often makes decisions for us. Providers may fail to share information we need about the benefits and burdens of treatment options. Partial understanding prevents truly informed consent for crucial treatment decisions.

Compassion & Choices is leading the way to transform our "conveyor belt" healthcare system, which promotes needless pain and suffering, into one where people are in charge of decisions that will affect quality of life as illnesses progress. We envision patient-driven processes that honor an individual's values, beliefs and priorities in life. We are working toward a system that supports decisions that reflect individual values, in candid consultation with doctors and loved ones. This includes decisions about dying with intention, if pain and suffering become too great.

Join the movement to create a society where, in Barbara Coombs Lee's words: "A good death is one that honors the life that's been lived."

Please visit CompassionAndChoices.org today and give as generously as you can, so together we can help bring peace of mind to people who want their wishes honored at the end of life.

275